Substance Abuse During Pregnancy

Editors

HILARY SMITH CONNERY
WILLIAM F. RAYBURN

OBSTETRICS AND GYNECOLOGY CLINICS OF NORTH AMERICA

www.obgyn.theclinics.com

Consulting Editor
WILLIAM F. RAYBURN

June 2014 • Volume 41 • Number 2

ELSEVIER

1600 John F. Kennedy Boulevard • Suite 1800 • Philadelphia, Pennsylvania, 19103-2899

http://www.theclinics.com

OBSTETRICS AND GYNECOLOGY CLINICS OF NORTH AMERICA Volume 41, Number 2
June 2014 ISSN 0889-8545, ISBN-13: 978-0-323-29926-8

Editor: Kerry Holland
Developmental Editor: Stephanie Carter

Obstetrics and Gynecology Clinics (ISSN 0889-8545) is published quarterly by Elsevier Inc., 360 Park Avenue South, New York, NY 10010-1710. Months of issue are March, June, September, and December. Periodicals postage paid at New York, NY, and additional mailing offices. Subscription price per year is $310.00 (US individuals), $545.00 (US institutions), $155.00 (US students), $370.00 (Canadian individuals), $688.00 (Canadian institutions), $225.00 (Canadian students), $450.00 (foreign individuals), $688.00 (foreign institutions), and $225.00 (foreign students). To receive student/resident rate, orders must be accompanied by name of affiliated institution, date of term, and the signature of program/residency coordinator on institution letterhead. Orders will be billed at individual rate until proof of status is received. Foreign air speed delivery is included in all *Clinics* subscription prices. All prices are subject to change without notice. POSTMASTER: Send address changes to *Obstetrics and Gynecology Clinics*, Elsevier Health Sciences Division, Subscription Customer Service, 3251 Riverport Lane, Maryland Heights, MO 63043. **Customer Service: Telephone: 1-800-654-2452 (U.S. and Canada); 314-447-8871 (outside U.S. and Canada). Fax: 314-447-8029. E-mail: journalscustomerservice-usa@elsevier.com (for print support); journalsonlinesupport-usa@elsevier. com (for online support).**

Reprints. For copies of 100 or more of articles in this publication, please contact the Commercial Reprints Department, Elsevier Inc., 360 Park Avenue South, New York, New York 10010-1710. Tel.: 212-633-3874; Fax: 212-633-3820; E-mail: reprints@elsevier.com.

Obstetrics and Gynecology Clinics of North America is also published in Spanish by McGraw-Hill Interamericana Editores S.A., P.O. Box 5-237, 06500, Mexico; in Portuguese by Reichmann and Affonso Editores, Rio de Janeiro, Brazil; and in Greek by Paschalidis Medical Publications, Athens, Greece.

Obstetrics and Gynecology Clinics of North America is covered in MEDLINE/PubMed (Index Medicus), Excerpta Medica, Current Concepts/Clinical Medicine, Science Citation Index, BIOSIS, CINAHL, and ISI/BIOMED.

Contributors

CONSULTING EDITOR

WILLIAM F. RAYBURN, MD, MBA
Division of Maternal Fetal Medicine, Professor and Chair, Department of Obstetrics and Gynecology; Associate Dean, Continuing Medical Education and Professional Development, University of New Mexico School of Medicine, Albuquerque, New Mexico

EDITORS

HILARY SMITH CONNERY, MD, PhD
Clinical Director, Division of Alcohol and Drug Abuse; Assistant Professor, Department of Psychiatry, Harvard Medical School, McLean Hospital, Belmont, Massachusetts

WILLIAM F. RAYBURN, MD, MBA
Division of Maternal Fetal Medicine, Professor and Chair, Department of Obstetrics and Gynecology; Associate Dean, Continuing Medical Education and Professional Development, University of New Mexico School of Medicine, Albuquerque, New Mexico

AUTHORS

BRITTANY B. ALBRIGHT, MD, MPH
Massachusetts General Hospital/McLean Hospital Adult Psychiatry Residency Program, Boston, Massachusetts

GRACE CHANG, MD, MPH
Professor of Psychiatry, Harvard Medical School, Boston; Department of Psychiatry, VA Boston Healthcare System, Brockton, Massachusetts

HILARY SMITH CONNERY, MD, PhD
Clinical Director, Division of Alcohol and Drug Abuse; Assistant Professor, Department of Psychiatry, Harvard Medical School, McLean Hospital, Belmont, Massachusetts

MEGAN DUFFY, BA
Department of Psychiatry and Behavioral Sciences, Johns Hopkins University School of Medicine, Baltimore, Maryland

SARAH GOPMAN, BA, MD
Assistant Professor, Family and Community Medicine, University of New Mexico, Albuquerque, New Mexico

SHELLY F. GREENFIELD, MD, MPH
Chief Academic Officer; Chief, Division of Women's Mental Health; Director, Clinical and Health Services Research and Education, Division of Alcohol and Drug Abuse, McLean Hospital, Belmont; Professor, Department of Psychiatry, Harvard Medical School, Boston, Massachusetts

NANCY A. HAUG, PhD
The Gronowski Center, Palo Alto University, Los Altos, California

BRADLEY D. HOLBROOK, MD
Division of Maternal-Fetal Medicine, Department of Obstetrics and Gynecology,
University of New Mexico School of Medicine, Albuquerque, New Mexico

ANDREW HSI, MD
Professor, Department of Pediatrics, University of New Mexico, Albuquerque, New Mexico

LUIS A. IZQUIERDO, MD, MBA
Associate Professor, Division of Maternal Fetal Medicine, University of New Mexico
School of Medicine, Albuquerque, New Mexico

LAWRENCE LEEMAN, MD, MPH
Professor, Departments of Family and Community Medicine, Obstetrics & Gynecology,
University of New Mexico, Albuquerque, New Mexico

MARY E. MCCAUL, PhD
Department of Psychiatry and Behavioral Sciences, Johns Hopkins University School of
Medicine, Baltimore, Maryland

R. KATHRYN MCHUGH, PhD
Assistant Professor, Division of Alcohol and Drug Abuse, McLean Hospital, Belmont;
Department of Psychiatry, Harvard Medical School, Boston, Massachusetts

MARJORIE MEYER, MD
Associate Professor, Maternal Fetal Medicine, University of Vermont, Burlington, Vermont

ELLEN L. MOZURKEWICH, MD, MS
Division of Maternal Fetal Medicine, Department of Obstetrics and Gynecology,
University of New Mexico School of Medicine, Albuquerque, New Mexico

SHARON PHELAN, MD, FACOG
Professor, Department of Obstetrics and Gynecology, University of New Mexico,
Albuquerque, New Mexico

WILLIAM F. RAYBURN, MD, MBA
Division of Maternal Fetal Medicine, Professor and Chair, Department of Obstetrics
and Gynecology; Associate Dean, Continuing Medical Education and Professional
Development, University of New Mexico School of Medicine, Albuquerque, New Mexico

JOHN M. RODOLICO, PhD
Program Director, Division of Child and Adolescent Psychiatry, Child and Adolescent
Psychiatry Residential Treatment, McLean Hospital, Belmont; Assistant Professor in
Clinical Psychology, Harvard Medical School, Boston, Massachusetts

MARY BETH SUTTER, MD
Maternal Child Health Fellow, Department of Family and Community Medicine, University
of New Mexico, Albuquerque, New Mexico

SARA WIGDERSON, BA
Clinical Research Assistant, Division of Alcohol and Drug Abuse; Division of Women's
Mental Health, McLean Hospital, Belmont, Massachusetts

NICOLE YONKE, MD, MPH
Assistant Professor, Division of Maternal Child Health, University of New Mexico School
of Medicine, Albuquerque, New Mexico

Contents

A significant number of women of reproductive age in the United States use addictive substances. In 2012 more than 50% reported current use of alcohol, 20% used tobacco products, and approximately 13% used other drugs. Among women, use of these substances is associated with several significant medical, psychiatric, and social consequences, and the course of illness may progress more rapidly in women than in men. The prevalence of substance use and evidence of accelerated illness progression in women highlight the importance of universal substance use screening in women in primary care settings.

Substance use among adolescents increases the risk of unplanned pregnancies, which then increases the risk of fetal exposure to addictive, teratogenic substances. Specific interventions are necessary to target pregnancy planning and contraception among reproductive-age substance users. Screening for substance use using the CRAFFT is recommended in all health care settings treating adolescent patients. Screening for tobacco and nicotine use is also recommended along with the provision of smoking cessation interventions. Using motivational interviewing style and strategies is recommended to engage adolescents in discussions related to reducing substance use, risky sexual behavior, and probability of unplanned pregnancy or late-detection pregnancy.

The use of alcohol and other substances is not infrequent during pregnancy and may be associated with adverse effects on pregnancy outcome. Many pregnant women may continue these practices throughout pregnancy and even after delivery, unless they are recognized and assessed. Screening may be one way to achieve consistent and early identification. Prenatal health care providers may wish to screen all pregnant patients for their use of alcohol and other drugs using an approach that works best in their setting. A positive screen is an opportunity for the clinician and patient to discuss health practices and behaviors.

The incidence of substance abuse in pregnancy is substantial and affects pregnancy health and outcomes. Multiple challenges exist in the identification of women with substance abuse disorders in pregnancy and the provision of care. A multidisciplinary approach has been shown to be most successful in providing comprehensive and effective care. This article outlines key aspects of prenatal and postpartum care, with a brief overview provided of intrapartum care. Issues covered include screening, opioid replacement therapy, comorbid medical and psychiatric conditions, environmental stressors, parenting preparation, pain management in labor and postpartum, breastfeeding guidance, prevention of relapse, and assistance with postpartum transition to primary care.

Substance use is prevalent in the United States, especially in the reproductive age population. Even though a reduction in substance use may occur during pregnancy, some women may not alter their drug use patterns until at least pregnancy is confirmed. For these reasons, a large number of fetuses are exposed to illicit substances, including during critical stages of organogenesis. Associating illicit drug use with eventual pregnancy outcome is difficult. This article presents issues pertaining to limitations with published investigations about fetal risks and describes the most current information in humans about fetal effects from specific illicit substances.

Buprenorphine and methadone are opioid-receptor agonists used as opioid substitution therapy during pregnancy to limit exposure of the fetus to cycles of opioid withdrawal and reduce the risk of infectious comorbidities of illicit opioid use. As part of a comprehensive care plan, such therapy may result in improved access to prenatal care, reduced illicit drug use, reduced exposure to infections associated with intravenous drug use, and improved maternal nutrition and infant birth weight. This article describes differences in patient selection between the two drugs, their relative safety during pregnancy, and changes in daily doses as a guide for prescribing clinicians.

More than 400,000 deaths occur per year in the United States that are attributable to cigarette smoking; the risks to the general public are widely known. The risk to women, especially those who are pregnant, is less commonly known. During pregnancy, smoking increases the risk of low birth weight infants, placental problems (previa and/or abruption), chronic hypertensive disorders, and fetal death. It is proposed that much of this happens because of vasoconstriction with decreased uterine blood flow from nicotine, carbon monoxide toxicity, and increased cyanide production. Infants of smoking mothers have increased risks, such as sudden infant death syndrome.

Women who use tobacco, alcohol and drugs during pregnancy are at increased risk of maternal and fetal morbidity. Universal screening using empirically validated approaches can improve identification of substance-using pregnant women and facilitate comprehensive assessment of treatment needs. There is strong evidence for effectiveness of psychosocial and behavioral substance abuse treatments across a range of intensities and levels of care. In addition to addressing substance use, services for co-occurring psychiatric disorders, trauma exposure, and prenatal care are important components of coordinated systems of care. More research on and greater access to evidence-based interventions is needed for this underserved population.

Chronic opioid therapy during pregnancy is perilous, but not simply because of neonatal effects: it is perilous because women are at particular risk for misprescription, misuse, dependence, overdose, and death. Opioids may be teratogens and should be avoided in the periconception period. Accidental childhood poisoning and purposeful teen experimentation are increased with opioid prescriptions in the home. Risks to pregnancy span the pre- and periconception period; neonatal risk following in utero opioid exposure is well documented. When the authors' patients request opioids for chronic pain, they care for them in a comprehensive and compassionate matter, which often will require therapeutic approaches other than chronic opioid therapy.

During early gestation, drugs have teratogenic effects and can be associated with structural anomalies in the fetus. Substance abuse can also have physiologic effects on the mother and fetus, including decreased uterine blood flow, increased vascular resistance, and an increase in fetal blood pressure. Women at increased risk for stillbirth should undergo antepartum fetal surveillance initiated at 32 weeks of gestation. Because of the high incidence of low birth weight, fetal anomalies, preterm delivery, and growth restriction in these patients, ultrasonography for appropriate pregnancy dating, a detailed anatomic survey, and cervical length should be performed at 20 weeks' gestation.

Neonatal opioid withdrawal syndrome is common due to the current opioid addiction epidemic. Infants born to women covertly abusing prescription opioids may not be identified as at risk until withdrawal signs present. Buprenorphine is a newer treatment for maternal opioid addiction and appears to result in a milder withdrawal syndrome than methadone. Initial treatment is with nonpharmacological measures including decreasing stimuli, however pharmacological treatment is commonly required. Opioid monotherapy is preferred, with phenobarbital or clonidine uncommonly needed as adjunctive therapy. Rooming-in and breastfeeding may decease the severity of withdrawal. Limited evidence is available regarding long-term effects of perinatal opioid exposure.

OBSTETRICS AND GYNECOLOGY CLINICS

ISSUE OF RELATED INTEREST

Perinatology Clinics, December 2012 (Vol. 39, Issue 4)
Resuscitation of the Fetus and Newborn
Praveen Kumar and Lou Halamek, *Editors*

NOW AVAILABLE FOR YOUR iPhone and iPad

Foreword
Substance Abuse During Pregnancy

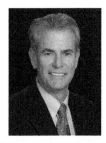

William F. Rayburn, MD, MBA
Consulting Editor

In 2003, Dr Michael Bogenschutz and I guest-edited an issue of *Obstetrics and Gynecology Clinics of North America* pertaining to "substance use disorders and women's health." That undertaking was in response to the misuse of illegal and controlled drugs, alcohol, and tobacco that became a more widely recognized national health problem. Although more frequent in men, substance use disorders (abuse and dependence) remained common in women, with overall lifetime prevalence estimated at nearly one in five women, excluding nicotine dependence.

In that issue, we asked the authors to characterize how substance misuse affected women and men differently. Substance-dependent women tended to suffer more severe medical and interpersonal consequences than men, and their dependence progressed more rapidly. Women with substance use disorders were reported to demonstrate different patterns of comorbid psychiatric illnesses, which in some cases played a role in the cause of their substance use disorder. Multiple barriers to effective diagnosis and treatment of substance use disorders were reported, including stigmatization of substance-using women, fear of loss of child custody, treatment programs designed for men, and a paucity of treatments, pharmacologic as well as psychosocial, that have been empirically validated in women.

Hopefully, these barriers have improved for all women, particularly those of reproductive age. Yet substance use continues to remain a major social and medical problem and women's substance use patterns are increasingly more similar to men's. The gap is narrowing, making this topic even more relevant now. For this reason, I chose to pursue an update issue of our *Obstetrics and Gynecology Clinics of North America* after more than a decade, which focused solely on ramifications of substance use and pregnancy. As physicians for women's health care, obstetricians play important, often frontline, roles in addressing substance use disorders. These roles may include screening patients for contraception and pregnancy, providing preventive education about substance use, advising patients about social and support groups, practicing

Obstet Gynecol Clin N Am 41 (2014) xi–xii
http://dx.doi.org/10.1016/j.ogc.2014.02.012
0889-8545/14/$ – see front matter © 2014 Elsevier Inc. All rights reserved.

safe prescription writing, undertaking fetal surveillance, and facilitating referrals for comanagement.

It is my pleasure to coedit this issue with the talents of Dr Hilary Smith Connery, a very capable psychiatrist trained in addiction medicine. Together, we attempted to provide relevant information to offer strategies for busy clinicians about providing more optimal and often interdisciplinary care of pregnant women with substance use problems. Our experienced and well-qualified team of authors hopes that practical evidence-based information provided herein will aid in the development and implementation of diagnostic and treatment programs for our needy patients and their families before and after the delivery of their babies.

William F. Rayburn, MD, MBA
Department of Obstetrics and Gynecology
Continuing Medical Education
and Professional Development
University of New Mexico School of Medicine
MSC10 5580, 1 University of New Mexico
Albuquerque, NM 87131-0001, USA

E-mail address:
wrayburn@salud.unm.edu

Preface

Substance Abuse During Pregnancy

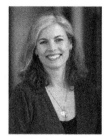 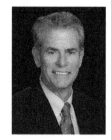

Hilary Smith Connery, MD, PhD   William F. Rayburn, MD, MBA
Editors

This issue of *Obstetrics and Gynecology Clinics of North America* deals with the timely subject of substance use during pregnancy. Alcohol, tobacco, and illicit drug use is prevalent among reproductive-age women. Even though a reduction in use often occurs during pregnancy, many women continue to use substances until a pregnancy is either actually diagnosed or well underway. Patient interviews and urine toxicologic testing at the initial prenatal visit and at delivery suggest that substance use during pregnancy ranges from 0.4% to 27%, depending on the population surveyed.

Care of the pregnant woman with a substance use disorder is often complex and demanding. Providers must be aware of these women's unique psychologic and social needs and the related legal and ethical ramifications surrounding pregnancy. In addition, effects from specific illicit drugs on eventual perinatal outcomes are difficult to predict. Concurrent use of multiple substances and co-occurring mental health problems are common. Many pregnant substance abusers are members of economically disadvantaged segments of society in which unfavorable perinatal outcomes are more common.

This issue consists of a well-qualified team of obstetricians-gynecologists, psychiatrists, and family physicians, focusing on various issues related directly to pregnancies complicated by substance use. Topics of interest include epidemiology and screening for hazardous and harmful substance use, teratogenic risks, psychiatric comorbidities, comprehensive treatment approaches before and after delivery, fetal surveillance, and team-based perinatal management. Particularly new information relates to prescribing buprenorphine, neonatal abstinence syndrome, and adolescent substance use.

Our intent is to activate attention to issues about substance use disorders for all providers caring for pregnant women and women of child-bearing age who may be at increased risk for unintended pregnancy due to substance use patterns. Practical information provided herein will hopefully offer strategies to optimize team-based care for this vulnerable population and their unborn infants. We are grateful to our friends

Obstet Gynecol Clin N Am 41 (2014) xiii–xiv
http://dx.doi.org/10.1016/j.ogc.2014.02.003
0889-8545/14/$ – see front matter © 2014 Published by Elsevier Inc.

obgyn.theclinics.com

and colleagues, who contributed their time and expertise to this edition. Their commitment to quality care and advancement of patient safety are exemplary.

Hilary Smith Connery, MD, PhD
Division of Alcohol and Drug Abuse
Department of Psychiatry
Harvard Medical School, McLean Hospital
115 Mill Street, Mail Stop 222
Belmont, MA 02478-1064, USA

William F. Rayburn, MD, MBA
Department of Obstetrics and Gynecology
Continuing Medical Education and Professional Development
University of New Mexico School of Medicine
MSC10 5580, 1 University of New Mexico
Albuquerque, NM 87131-0001, USA

E-mail addresses:
hconnery@mclean.harvard.edu (H.S. Connery)
wrayburn@salud.unm.edu (W.F. Rayburn)

Epidemiology of Substance Use in Reproductive-Age Women

R. Kathryn McHugh, PhD[a,b], Sara Wigderson, BA[a,c],
Shelly F. Greenfield, MD, MPH[a,b,c],*

KEYWORDS

- Substance use • Substance use disorders • Women • Pregnancy

KEY POINTS

- Gender differences in the prevalence of substance use are declining, with women comprising a growing percentage of those who use addictive substances.
- Alcohol, nicotine, and drug use are common in women of reproductive age and problem-level use of addictive substances is associated with several medical, psychiatric, and social consequences.
- The high prevalence of substance use in pregnant women highlights the importance of improving public education on the risks of substance use in pregnancy, increasing preventive services, and providing addiction treatment for those pregnant women in need.

Although the prevalence of use of addictive substances is greater in men than in women, this gender gap is steadily narrowing in the United States and internationally.[1,2] In 2012, of the almost 41.5 million individuals in the United States who reported using illicit drugs in the previous year, more than 42% were women.[3] Women represented more than 40% of users of tobacco products (33 million women) and almost 50% of alcohol users (85.5 million women).[3] During this same time, more than 7.6 million women ages 12 and older in the United States were estimated to suffer from a substance use disorder.[3]

An increase in research on substance use in women in recent years has found that women may be more susceptible to the medical, psychiatric, and social consequences of addictive substances than men. Relative to men, women exhibit a shorter

Disclosures: Drs R.K. McHugh and S.F. Greenfield and Ms S. Wigderson have no relevant conflicts of interest to disclose.
[a] Division of Alcohol and Drug Abuse, McLean Hospital, 115 Mill Street, Belmont, MA 02478, USA; [b] Department of Psychiatry, Harvard Medical School, 25 Shattuck Street, Boston, MA 02115, USA; [c] Division of Women's Mental Health, McLean Hospital, 115 Mill Street, Belmont, MA 02478, USA
* Corresponding author. McLean Hospital, Proctor House 3, MS 222, 115 Mill Street, Belmont, MA 02478.
E-mail address: sgreenfield@mclean.harvard.edu

latency from the initiation of substance use to the onset and progression of substance use disorders (a "telescoping" course of illness).[4,5] Moreover, when women present for treatment of substance use disorders, they often report greater impairment relative to men in employment, social, psychiatric, and medical domains.[6,7] Women with substance use disorders also disproportionately suffer from cooccurring anxiety and depressive disorders[4,8] and may be more likely to use substances to manage negative affect.[7,9] In pregnant women, substance use is a particular concern for the health of the developing fetus due to the teratogenic effects of several addictive substances,[10] as well as negative effects on fetal development via poor maternal health and health behaviors (eg, nutrition).[11]

This article provides a brief overview of the epidemiology of alcohol, nicotine, and illicit substance use in women of reproductive age including prevalence, medical consequences, and treatment considerations. **Box 1** lists key definitions.

ALCOHOL USE
Prevalence and Course

In 2012, 47.9% of American women ages 12 years and over reported that they were current alcohol users.[12] Among women ages 14 to 44 who were not pregnant, 55.5% reported alcohol use, 24.7% reported binge drinking, and 5.2% reported binge drinking on at least 5 days in the past month.[12] These prevalence estimates use

---

Box 1
Key definitions

Substance use

The consumption of any psychoactive substance, including alcohol, nicotine, and illicit drugs, and nonmedical use of prescription drugs.

Substance use disorder

A pattern of use of an addictive substance that is associated with significant impairment and/or distress as indicated by symptoms such as disruption of important life obligations, the inability to reduce use, and physiologic tolerance for the substance. The prevalence estimates reported in this article correspond to the diagnoses of substance abuse (requiring 1 of 4 symptoms) and substance dependence (requiring 3 of 7 symptoms) as defined by the *Diagnostic and Statistical Manual of Mental Disorders, 4th Edition* (*DSM-IV*). The recently published *DSM-5* collapses these into a single disorder and includes minor modifications to the list of possible symptoms (requiring 2 of 11 symptoms), and thus these prevalence estimates will likely change as studies begin to use this new classification system.

Binge drinking

A pattern of alcohol consumption that brings the blood-alcohol-concentration level to 0.08% or more. This pattern of drinking usually corresponds to 5 or more drinks on a single occasion for men or 4 or more drinks on a single occasion for women, generally within about 2 hours.

Heavy or "At-Risk" Drinking

For women: more than 3 drinks on any single day or more than 7 drinks per week. For men: more than 4 drinks on any single day or more than 14 drinks per week.

Nonmedical prescription drug use

Use of a prescribed medication at either a higher dose or a greater frequency than prescribed, or use of medication without a prescription.

Data from Refs.[98–101]

definitions of binge drinking established by the Substance Abuse and Mental Health Services Administration[12]; however, these likely are underestimates because these definitions rely on a higher threshold for women than the widely accepted definitions used by the National Institute on Alcohol Abuse and Alcoholism (NIAAA) (see **Box 1**). The prevalence of alcohol use disorders in women is approximately 4.9% in the past year and 19.5% lifetime.[12]

Alcohol use typically is initiated in late adolescence and problematic use is most prevalent in young adulthood for both men and women. Most (more than 80%) individuals first using alcohol in 2012 were younger than 21, and more than 58% were younger than 18, with similar numbers of initiators among men and women.[3] In addition to the overall increase in alcohol use in young women, binge drinking among young women has increased; 33.2% of women aged 18 to 25 reported binge drinking in the previous year.[3] Currently, 1 of every 8 U.S. women (nearly 14 million) binge drinks approximately 3 times each month with an average of 6 drinks per binge. The increase in binge drinking in young women prompted an alert from the Center for Disease Control and Prevention in January 2013 stating that binge drinking is a serious, underrecognized problem among women and girls.[13]

Medical Consequences

Alcohol-related medical complications are the eighth leading cause of death worldwide.[14] The NIAAA defines "low-risk" drinking for men as no more than 4 standard drinks in a day and no more than 14 drinks per week. For women, low-risk drinking is defined as no more than 3 standard drinks in a day and no more than 7 standard drinks per week.[15] A standard drink is the equivalent of a 12-oz. beer, a 5-oz. glass of wine, or 1.5 oz. of liquor. Heavy drinking in women is associated with greater mortality and shorter lifespan.[16,17] In addition to risks related to injury, heavy alcohol use has a wide range of negative effects on health, such as adverse effects on cognitive and immune functioning, and increased risk for hypertension, cardiovascular and gastrointestinal disease, and the development of certain cancers including breast, mouth, and throat cancer.[18] Binge drinking is also associated with injuries and risky behaviors,[19] and greater susceptibility to sexual victimization and violence.[20,21] In addition, binge drinking is associated with unintended pregnancy and sexually transmitted diseases, such as HIV.[19,22]

Pregnant Women

Although the prevalence of alcohol use in pregnant women is lower than in nonpregnant women, in 2012 among pregnant women ages 14 to 44, 8.5% reported alcohol use, 2.7% reported binge drinking, and 0.3% reported binge drinking on at least 5 of 30 days during pregnancy.[12] Among pregnant women ages 18 to 50, 3.6% met diagnostic criteria for an alcohol use disorder.[23]

Alcohol crosses the placenta and is a well-established teratogen.[24] Fetal alcohol spectrum disorders (FASDs), conditions associated with irreversible birth defects, are among the most concerning potential consequences of alcohol use in pregnancy. The most severe disorder within this spectrum is fetal alcohol syndrome, which includes mental and physical defects, such as abnormal facial features, growth deficits, and problems with the central nervous system.[25] Other FASDs are characterized by a range of problems, such as deficits in intellect and learning and damage to organs and physical features.[26] The overall prevalence of FASDs is estimated to be approximately 2% to 5% of births.[27]

Although low levels of drinking during pregnancy have not been associated with growth abnormalities,[28] even low levels of use have been associated with behavioral problems.[29] Research in animals suggests that even light to moderate alcohol exposure throughout gestation has negative effects on development.[30,31] Several imaging studies in humans have demonstrated that prenatal alcohol exposure disrupts development of both gray and white matter and illustrate alcohol-related alterations in cerebral blood flow, neurotransmitters, and neuronal activity; individuals with prenatal alcohol exposure can exhibit neuronal anomalies and dysfunction without distinct facial dysmorphology.[32] Given the range of adverse alcohol effects on fetal development demonstrated by current research, the U.S. Surgeon General has recommended that women abstain from alcohol consumption during pregnancy.[33]

The effect of alcohol use on breast-feeding infants has been less well studied; however, studies suggest that a small percentage of alcohol consumed is absorbed in breast milk and passed to the infant during breast-feeding.[34] Alcohol use has been shown to inhibit lactation and result in modified feeding patterns by the infant[35,36] as well as other potential adverse effects on gross motor development and early learning.[35] Other research on the effects of alcohol exposure during breast-feeding on the infant has yielded inconsistent findings.[37] However, alcohol inhibits lactation and no safe levels of alcohol consumption while breast feeding have been established with regard to transmission to the infant.

NICOTINE USE
Prevalence and Course

Despite steady decreases in tobacco product use in the United States over the past 10 years, use remains high. In 2012, 20.9% of women aged 12 and older reported use of tobacco products. During this time, the female-to-male ratio was 1 to 1.6, and almost equivalent among female and male adolescents (6.3% vs 6.8%).[12] Cigarette smoking remains the most common method of tobacco use, and most (more than 60%) cigarette smokers are daily smokers, with more than 40% smoking a pack or more per day.[12]

Tobacco use often is initiated during adolescence. In 2012, more than 50% of first-time smokers were younger than 18.[12] The likelihood of transitioning from use to dependence is exceptionally high for nicotine, with estimates that more than 67% of nicotine users will develop nicotine dependence at some time during their life.[38] Although several risk factors have been identified for smoking in both genders, such as parent and peer smoking and low socioeconomic status, women may be disproportionately affected by weight-related and affect-related risk factors. Adolescent women who report weight-related and diet-related concerns seem to escalate to regular smoking more quickly than those who do not,[39] and women report postcessation weight gain as a barrier to quitting more commonly than men.[40] Women also report higher distress and urges to smoke in response to negative affective states.[9] Timing of quit attempts with menstrual cycle phase may also be important for women, because there is some evidence that women achieve greater success rates when smoking cessation efforts are timed in the follicular rather than the luteal phase of the menstrual cycle.[41]

Medical Consequences

Smoking is the leading preventable cause of death in the United States,[42] and the second leading cause of mortality worldwide.[14] Cigarette smoking has several significant health consequences for women, such as morbidity and mortality associated with cardiovascular disease,[43] respiratory disease,[44] and a range of cancers including lung, throat, breast, and ovarian cancer.[45-49]

Despite some evidence that women are more susceptible to the carcinogenic effects of cigarette smoking than men, several large studies have suggested that the incidence of lung cancer among smokers is equivalent between men and women.[45] Lung cancer is the second most common cancer in women and the leading cause of cancer death in women.[50] Smoking has been estimated to cause 80% of lung cancer deaths in women, and smokers are 15 to 30 times more likely to develop lung cancer relative to nonsmokers.[50] Heavy, long-term smoking appears to increase the risk for breast cancer[48] and doubles the risk of developing ovarian cancer.[49]

Pregnant Women

In a 2012 study, 15.9% of pregnant women between the ages of 15 and 44 reported smoking cigarettes in the previous month.[12] Importantly, although the prevalence of cigarette smoking in nonpregnant women in this age group has decreased in the past 10 years, the prevalence of cigarette smoking in pregnant women has remained relatively stable.[12] Women with greater severity of nicotine dependence, a partner who also smokes, and greater socioeconomic stress may have greater difficulty with abstaining from smoking during pregnancy.[51]

The teratogenic effects of smoking have been widely documented. Nicotine, as well as several other harmful compounds in cigarette smoke, crosses the placenta and has wide-ranging negative effects on fetal development. Smoking during pregnancy has been associated with low birth weight, being small for gestational age, and preterm birth,[52,53] as well as long-term effects on cognition.[54] Smoking cessation can lead to significant reductions in these health risks for both women[55] and the developing fetus (particularly quitting in the first trimester).[56]

ILLICIT DRUG USE AND NONMEDICAL PRESCRIPTION DRUG USE
Prevalence and Course

The gaps between men and women in prevalence remain highest for illicit drugs relative to other addictive substances.[12] However, women and men exhibit a similar prevalence of nonmedical prescription drug use and prescription drug use disorders,[57,58] and the prevalence of these problems (particularly with opioid analgesics) has increased rapidly over the past 15 years.[59] Approximately 13% of women in the United States use illicit drugs or nonprescribed drugs each year and more than 43% will engage in drug use in their lifetime.[3]

Marijuana is the most commonly used illicit drug among both men and women (38.1% of women aged 12 and older report lifetime use of marijuana), followed by nonmedical use of prescription medications (18.9%), cocaine and hallucinogens (approximately 11% each), inhalants (5.3%), and heroin (1.0%).[3]

Although many women who use illicit or nonprescribed drugs will not develop substance use disorders, it is estimated that approximately 8% to 9% of marijuana users will develop marijuana dependence in their lifetime,[38] and 5% to 6% of first-time cocaine users will develop cocaine dependence within a year (up to 16% within 10 years).[60] Nonmedical prescription drug use is associated with later development of a substance use disorder, particularly among younger users.[61] Approximately 1.2% of women met the criteria for a drug use disorder in the past year and 7.1% over the course of their lifetime.[62] Including both men and women, the prevalence of illicit drug use disorders is highest among those ages 18 to 25 (7.8%) relative to those younger than 18 (4%) and those 26 and older (1.8%).[3]

Medical Consequences

The use of illicit substances and nonmedical use of prescription drugs are associated with a myriad of significant health consequences, such as negative effects on cognition, increased risk for infectious disease, respiratory and cardiovascular illnesses, and accidental overdose.

Although it has been far less studied than tobacco, marijuana smoking (particularly heavy use) appears to be associated with respiratory illness, such as impairment of airway function[63] and risk for lung cancer.[64] Moreover, many marijuana users also are regular users of nicotine, and the use of both substances may confer particularly elevated risk for respiratory illness, such as chronic obstructive pulmonary disease.[65] Marijuana use—particularly beginning in early adolescence—may have significant negative effects on cognition, such as lower intelligence and greater impulsivity.[66,67] In addition to these adverse medical consequences, a prospective longitudinal study demonstrated that marijuana use in adolescence, especially use before age 15, conferred an elevated risk for developing schizophrenia in adulthood.[68]

Cocaine use has significant medical consequences and is associated with more emergency room visits than any other addictive drug.[69] Cocaine is associated with substantial cardiovascular risks, such as myocardial infarction, cardiac arrhythmias, and hypertension,[70] as well as deleterious effects on the pulmonary and central nervous systems.[71,72] Research has identified several gender differences in behavioral and neurobehavioral responses to cocaine, which may be mediated by gonadal hormones.[73]

Opioids also are associated with several medical consequences, such as accidental overdose and risks associated with intravenous drug administration. Among the most concerning risks are infectious diseases associated with shared injection equipment, such as HIV and hepatitis C. Women with substance use disorders may be more susceptible to risky injection behaviors and risky sexual behaviors.[74,75] Accidental overdose deaths from prescription opioids increased dramatically in the United States in the 2000s and have the highest mortality prevalence, followed by cocaine, sedative hypnotics, and heroin.[76]

Pregnant Women

Estimates of illicit drug use among pregnant women suggest that the annual prevalence of use (approximately 6%) is lower than in nonpregnant women.[12] Prevalence is highest among young pregnant women (18.3% among women aged 15–17 and 3.4% among those 26–44).[12] Approximately 1.6% of pregnant women meet the criteria for a drug use disorder.[23] Marijuana and cocaine appear to be the most commonly used illicit drugs among pregnant women[77]; however, in certain geographic areas (eg, the Western United States), methamphetamine use is a significant problem among pregnant women and is a common reason for seeking substance abuse treatment.[78]

Addictive illicit and prescription drugs are associated with several negative effects on fetal development. For example, exposure to marijuana,[79] cocaine,[80] and opioids[81] has been associated with growth restriction and low birth weight, poor neonatal outcomes,[82] and long-term negative effects on cognitive and academic performance in children.[83] Opioid use during pregnancy is associated with neonatal abstinence syndrome, a withdrawal syndrome that has been increasing in prevalence.[84]

A criticism of the relatively limited research on the effects of use of illicit drugs during pregnancy is that many studies have failed to control adequately for related factors that may contribute to poor outcomes, such as poverty, poor nutrition, and chronic stress. For example, prenatal cocaine exposure gained significant media attention in the 1980s due to the purported "crack-baby" epidemic. Although the use of cocaine during pregnancy is associated with several negative outcomes, many early reports of the severity of these effects were likely overstated. Recent studies controlling for other variables, such as poverty, have suggested that cocaine-exposed children exhibit similar outcomes to those not exposed to cocaine—particularly when provided with early enrichment interventions.[85,86] Nonetheless, numerous studies suggest direct or indirect effects (eg, risk behaviors, poor maternal health) of illicit substance use on fetal development and outcomes, highlighting the importance of treatment in this population.

CLINICAL IMPLICATIONS: TREATMENT AND PREVENTION

Given the high prevalence of substance use in women, screening is critical to the early identification of problematic use and substance use disorders. Screening and brief interventions implemented in primary care settings including general medicine, obstetrics and gynecologic services, and pediatric and adolescent medicine practices are effective for reducing problem use among women (including pregnant women).[87,88] Although there are several effective treatments for substance use disorders, less than 20% of women who need treatment receive it in a given year,[89] and women are less likely than men to engage in substance use disorder treatment.[57,90] This discrepancy may be attributable to barriers that disproportionately affect women, such as economic barriers, social stigma, cooccurring psychiatric disorders, and lack of child care.[90] Nonetheless, once in treatment, women and men have similar rates of treatment response.[7,91]

Among pregnant women, perception of risk appears to be a predictor of use,[92,93] highlighting the importance of education on the risks of substance use during pregnancy. Nonetheless, some women will have difficulty discontinuing substance use during pregnancy, such as those with substance use disorders. As treatment has been shown to improve the likelihood of quitting[87,94] and earlier discontinuation of substance use may decrease some risks to the woman and the developing fetus,[56] adequate screening and referral to services can be of particular benefit.

For pregnant women with more severe substance use disorders for which pharmacotherapy may be indicated, the balance between risk and benefit must be considered. Although opioid agonist therapies, such as methadone maintenance or buprenorphine maintenance therapy, continue to expose the fetus to the drug, the benefits of engaging in these therapies substantially outweigh the risks associated with continued illicit opioid use (eg, injection use, exposure to higher levels of drug, overdose risk) and provide significant advantage because of the association with better prenatal care and maternal and neonatal outcomes.[95–97]

SUMMARY

The use of alcohol, nicotine, and illicit and prescribed drugs is prevalent among women of reproductive age. Problem-level use of these substances is associated with several significant health consequences, and women may be particularly susceptible to a rapid progression from initial use of substances, to substance use disorders, to substantial impairment related to these disorders. Substance use disorders are common among women over their lifetime; however, women are less likely to receive substance use disorder care then men.

Substance use in pregnancy is a significant concern given the adverse health consequences for both the mother and the developing fetus. However, the prevalence of substance use among pregnant women continues to be a clinical and public health concern, with more than 1 in 10 pregnant women reporting alcohol or nicotine use, and 1 in 20 reporting other drug use, despite guidance from major groups such as the U.S. Surgeon General and the American Academy of Pediatrics urging abstinence from addictive substances during pregnancy. The evaluation of alcohol, nicotine, and other drug use in reproductive-aged women is critically important to identify harmful and hazardous use and to provide women with information on the risks of use, and brief interventions or referrals to substance use treatment as clinically indicated.

ACKNOWLEDGMENTS

The authors acknowledge National Institute on Drug Abuse grants K24 DA019855 (S.F.G.) and U10 DA015831 (S.F.G, R.K.M.).

REFERENCES

1. Keyes KM, Grant BF, Hasin DS. Evidence for a closing gender gap in alcohol use, abuse, and dependence in the United States population. Drug Alcohol Depend 2008;93:21–9.
2. Steingrimsson S, Carlsen HK, Sigfusson S, et al. The changing gender gap in substance use disorder: a total population-based study of psychiatric in-patients. Addiction 2012;107:1957–62.
3. Substance Abuse and Mental Health Services Administration. Results from the 2012 National Survey on Drug Use and Health: detailed tables. Rockville (MD): Substance Abuse and Mental Health Services Administration; 2013.
4. Khan SS, Secades-Villa R, Okuda M, et al. Gender differences in cannabis use disorders: results from the National Epidemiologic Survey of Alcohol and Related Conditions. Drug Alcohol Depend 2013;130:101–8.
5. Randall CL, Roberts JS, Del Boca FK, et al. Telescoping of landmark events associated with drinking: a gender comparison. J Stud Alcohol 1999;60: 252–60.
6. Hernandez-Avila CA, Rounsaville BJ, Kranzler HR. Opioid-, cannabis- and alcohol-dependent women show more rapid progression to substance abuse treatment. Drug Alcohol Depend 2004;74:265–72.
7. McHugh RK, Devito EE, Dodd D, et al. Gender differences in a clinical trial for prescription opioid dependence. J Subst Abuse Treat 2013;45:38–43.
8. Khan S, Okuda M, Hasin DS, et al. Gender differences in lifetime alcohol dependence: results from the national epidemiologic survey on alcohol and related conditions. Alcohol Clin Exp Res 2013;37:1696–705.
9. Saladin ME, Gray KM, Carpenter MJ, et al. Gender differences in craving and cue reactivity to smoking and negative affect/stress cues. Am J Addict 2012; 21:210–20.
10. Behnke M, Smith VC. Prenatal substance abuse: short- and long-term effects on the exposed fetus. Pediatrics 2013;131:e1009–24.
11. Knight EM, James H, Edwards CH, et al. Relationships of serum illicit drug concentrations during pregnancy to maternal nutritional status. J Nutr 1994;124: 973S–80S.
12. Substance Abuse and Mental Health Services Administration. Results from the 2012 National Survey on Drug Use and Health: summary of national findings, NSDUH Series H-46, HHS Publication No. (SMA) 13–4795. Rockville (MD): Substance Abuse and Mental Health Services Administration; 2013.

13. Binge drinking: a serious, under-recognized problem among women and girls. 2013. Available at: http://www.cdc.gov/VitalSigns/BingeDrinkingFemale/index.html. Accessed July 16, 2013.
14. World Health Organization. Global health risks: mortality and burden of disease attributable to selected major risks. Geneva (Switzerland): World Health Organization; 2009.
15. National Institute on Alcohol Abuse and Alcoholism. Helping patients who drink too much: a clinician's guide. Rockville (MD): National Institute on Alcohol Abuse and Alcoholism; 2007. NIH Publication No 07-3769.
16. Plunk AD, Syed-Mohammed H, Cavazos-Rehg P, et al. Alcohol consumption, heavy drinking, and mortality: rethinking the J-shaped curve. Alcohol Clin Exp Res 2014;38(2):471–8.
17. Smith EM, Cloninger CR, Bradford S. Predictors of mortality in alcoholic women: prospective follow-up study. Alcohol Clin Exp Res 1983;7:237–43.
18. National Institute on Alcohol Abuse and Alcoholism. Beyond hangovers: understanding alcohol's impact on health. NIH Publication No. 13-7604. Rockville (MD): National Institute on Alcohol Abuse and Alcoholism; 2010.
19. Wechsler H, Davenport A, Dowdall G, et al. Health and behavioral consequences of binge drinking in college. A national survey of students at 140 campuses. JAMA 1994;272:1672–7.
20. McCauley JL, Calhoun KS, Gidycz CA. Binge drinking and rape: a prospective examination of college women with a history of previous sexual victimization. J Interpers Violence 2010;25:1655–68.
21. Stappenbeck CA, Fromme K. A longitudinal investigation of heavy drinking and physical dating violence in men and women. Addict Behav 2010;35:479–85.
22. Naimi TS, Lipscomb LE, Brewer RD, et al. Binge drinking in the preconception period and the risk of unintended pregnancy: implications for women and their children. Pediatrics 2003;111:1136–41.
23. Vesga-Lopez O, Blanco C, Keyes K, et al. Psychiatric disorders in pregnant and postpartum women in the United States. Arch Gen Psychiatry 2008;65:805–15.
24. Warren KR, Foudin LL. Alcohol-related birth defects–the past, present, and future. Alcohol Res Health 2001;25:153–8.
25. Jones KL, Smith DW, Ulleland CN, et al. Pattern of malformation in offspring of chronic alcoholic mothers. Lancet 1973;1:1267–71.
26. Fetal alcohol spectrum disorders, facts about FASDs. 2011. Available at: http://www.cdc.gov/ncbddd/fasd/facts.html. Accessed December 13, 2013.
27. May PA, Gossage JP, Kalberg WO, et al. Prevalence and epidemiologic characteristics of FASD from various research methods with an emphasis on recent in-school studies. Dev Disabil Res Rev 2009;15:176–92.
28. Bakker R, Pluimgraaff LE, Steegers EA, et al. Associations of light and moderate maternal alcohol consumption with fetal growth characteristics in different periods of pregnancy: the Generation R Study. Int J Epidemiol 2010;39:777–89.
29. Sood B, Delaney-Black V, Covington C, et al. Prenatal alcohol exposure and childhood behavior at age 6 to 7 years: I. Dose-response effect. Pediatrics 2001;108:E34.
30. Probyn ME, Zanini S, Ward LC, et al. A rodent model of low- to moderate-dose ethanol consumption during pregnancy: patterns of ethanol consumption and effects on fetal and offspring growth. Reprod Fertil Dev 2012;24:859–70.
31. Vaglenova J, Petkov VV. Fetal alcohol effects in rats exposed pre- and postnatally to a low dose of ethanol. Alcohol Clin Exp Res 1998;22:697–703.

32. Thomas JD, Warren KR, Hewitt BG. Fetal alcohol spectrum disorders: from research to policy. Alcohol Res Health 2010;33:118–26.
33. Carmona RH. Alcohol warning for pregnant women. FDA Consum 2005;39(3):4.
34. Lawton ME. Alcohol in breast milk. Aust N Z J Obstet Gynaecol 1985;25:71–3.
35. Mennella JA. Short-term effects of maternal alcohol consumption on lactational performance. Alcohol Clin Exp Res 1998;22:1389–92.
36. Mennella JA. Regulation of milk intake after exposure to alcohol in mothers' milk. Alcohol Clin Exp Res 2001;25:590–3.
37. Haastrup MB, Pottegard A, Damkier P. Alcohol and breastfeeding. Basic Clin Pharmacol Toxicol 2014;114:168–73.
38. Lopez-Quintero C, Perez de los Cobos J, Hasin DS, et al. Probability and predictors of transition from first use to dependence on nicotine, alcohol, cannabis, and cocaine: results of the National Epidemiologic Survey on Alcohol and Related Conditions (NESARC). Drug Alcohol Depend 2011;115:120–30.
39. Blitstein JL, Robinson LA, Murray DM, et al. Rapid progression to regular cigarette smoking among nonsmoking adolescents: interactions with gender and ethnicity. Prev Med 2003;36:455–63.
40. Levine MD, Bush T, Magnusson B, et al. Smoking-related weight concerns and obesity: differences among normal weight, overweight, and obese smokers using a telephone tobacco quitline. Nicotine Tob Res 2013;15:1136–40.
41. Carpenter MJ, Saladin ME, Leinbach AS, et al. Menstrual phase effects on smoking cessation: a pilot feasibility study. J Womens Health (Larchmt) 2008;17:293–301.
42. Danaei G, Ding EL, Mozaffarian D, et al. The preventable causes of death in the United States: comparative risk assessment of dietary, lifestyle, and metabolic risk factors. PLoS Med 2009;6:e1000058.
43. Willett WC, Green A, Stampfer MJ, et al. Relative and absolute excess risks of coronary heart disease among women who smoke cigarettes. N Engl J Med 1987;317:1303–9.
44. U.S. Department of Health and Human Services. The health consequences of smoking: a report of the Surgeon General. Atlanta (GA): U.S. Department of Health and Human Services, Centers for Disease Control and Prevention, National Center for Chronic Disease Prevention and Health Promotion, Office on Smoking and Health; 2004.
45. Freedman ND, Leitzmann MF, Hollenbeck AR, et al. Cigarette smoking and subsequent risk of lung cancer in men and women: analysis of a prospective cohort study. Lancet Oncol 2008;9:649–56.
46. Freedman ND, Silverman DT, Hollenbeck AR, et al. Association between smoking and risk of bladder cancer among men and women. JAMA 2011;306:737–45.
47. Powell HA, Iyen-Omofoman B, Hubbard RB, et al. The association between smoking quantity and lung cancer in men and women. Chest 2013;143:123–9.
48. Gaudet MM, Gapstur SM, Sun J, et al. Active smoking and breast cancer risk: original cohort data and meta-analysis. J Natl Cancer Inst 2013;105:515–25.
49. Jordan SJ, Whiteman DC, Purdie DM, et al. Does smoking increase risk of ovarian cancer? A systematic review. Gynecol Oncol 2006;103:1122–9.
50. U.S. Cancer Statistics Working Group. United States cancer statistics: 1999-2010 incidence and mortality web-based report. Atlanta (GA): US Department of Health and Human Services, Centers for Disease Control and Prevention and National Cancer Institute; 2013.

51. Ma Y, Goins KV, Pbert L, et al. Predictors of smoking cessation in pregnancy and maintenance postpartum in low-income women. Matern Child Health J 2005;9: 393–402.
52. Ko TJ, Tsai LY, Chu LC, et al. Parental smoking during pregnancy and its association with low birth weight, small for gestational age, and preterm birth offspring: a birth cohort study. Pediatr Neonatol 2014;55(1):20–7.
53. Pollack H, Lantz PM, Frohna JG. Maternal smoking and adverse birth outcomes among singletons and twins. Am J Public Health 2000;90:395–400.
54. Chen R, Clifford A, Lang L, et al. Is exposure to secondhand smoke associated with cognitive parameters of children and adolescents?: a systematic literature review. Ann Epidemiol 2013;23:652–61.
55. Reichert V, Xue X, Bartscherer D, et al. A pilot study to examine the effects of smoking cessation on serum markers of inflammation in women at risk for cardiovascular disease. Chest 2009;136:212–9.
56. Polakowski LL, Akinbami LJ, Mendola P. Prenatal smoking cessation and the risk of delivering preterm and small-for-gestational-age newborns. Obstet Gynecol 2009;114:318–25.
57. Back SE, Payne RL, Simpson AN, et al. Gender and prescription opioids: findings from the National Survey on Drug Use and Health. Addict Behav 2010;35: 1001–7.
58. Parsells Kelly J, Cook SF, Kaufman DW, et al. Prevalence and characteristics of opioid use in the US adult population. Pain 2008;138:507–13.
59. Blanco C, Alderson D, Ogburn E, et al. Changes in the prevalence of non-medical prescription drug use and drug use disorders in the United States: 1991-1992 and 2001-2002. Drug Alcohol Depend 2007;90:252–60.
60. Wagner FA, Anthony JC. From first drug use to drug dependence: developmental periods of risk for dependence upon marijuana, cocaine, and alcohol. Neuropsychopharmacology 2002;26:479–88.
61. McCabe SE, West BT, Morales M, et al. Does early onset of non-medical use of prescription drugs predict subsequent prescription drug abuse and dependence? Results from a national study. Addiction 2007;102:1920–30.
62. Compton WM, Thomas YF, Stinson FS, et al. Prevalence, correlates, disability, and comorbidity of DSM-IV drug abuse and dependence in the United States: results from the National Epidemiologic Survey on Alcohol and Related Conditions. Arch Gen Psychiatry 2007;64:566–76.
63. Aldington S, Williams M, Nowitz M, et al. Effects of cannabis on pulmonary structure, function and symptoms. Thorax 2007;62:1058–63.
64. Callaghan RC, Allebeck P, Sidorchuk A. Marijuana use and risk of lung cancer: a 40-year cohort study. Cancer Causes Control 2013;24:1811–20.
65. Tan WC, Lo C, Jong A, et al. Marijuana and chronic obstructive lung disease: a population-based study. CMAJ 2009;180:814–20.
66. Gruber SA, Dahlgren MK, Sagar KA, et al. Worth the wait: effects of age of onset of marijuana use on white matter and impulsivity. Psychopharmacology (Berl) 2013. [Epub ahead of print].
67. Meier MH, Caspi A, Ambler A, et al. Persistent cannabis users show neuropsychological decline from childhood to midlife. Proc Natl Acad Sci U S A 2012; 109:E2657–64.
68. Arseneault L, Cannon M, Poulton R, et al. Cannabis use in adolescence and risk for adult psychosis: longitudinal prospective study. BMJ 2002;325:1212–3.
69. Substance Abuse and Mental Health Services Administration. Drug Abuse Warning Network, 2011. Rockville (MD): National Estimates of Drug-Related

Emergency Department Visits; 2013. HHS Publication No. (SMA) 13-4760. DAWN Series D-39.

70. Pozner CN, Levine M, Zane R. The cardiovascular effects of cocaine. J Emerg Med 2005;29:173–8.

71. de Almeida RR, de Souza LS, Mancano AD, et al. High-resolution computed tomographic findings of cocaine-induced pulmonary disease: a state of the art review. Lung 2014. [Epub ahead of print].

72. Franklin TR, Acton PD, Maldjian JA, et al. Decreased gray matter concentration in the insular, orbitofrontal, cingulate, and temporal cortices of cocaine patients. Biol Psychiatry 2002;51:134–42.

73. Evans SM, Foltin RW. Does the response to cocaine differ as a function of sex or hormonal status in human and non-human primates? Horm Behav 2010;58:13–21.

74. Brooks A, Meade CS, Potter JS, et al. Gender differences in the rates and correlates of HIV risk behaviors among drug abusers. Subst Use Misuse 2010;45: 2444–69.

75. Frajzyngier V, Neaigus A, Gyarmathy VA, et al. Gender differences in injection risk behaviors at the first injection episode. Drug Alcohol Depend 2007;89: 145–52.

76. Calcaterra S, Glanz J, Binswanger IA. National trends in pharmaceutical opioid related overdose deaths compared to other substance related overdose deaths: 1999-2009. Drug Alcohol Depend 2013;131:263–70.

77. Ebrahim SH, Gfroerer J. Pregnancy-related substance use in the United States during 1996-1998. Obstet Gynecol 2003;101:374–9.

78. Terplan M, Smith EJ, Kozloski MJ, et al. Methamphetamine use among pregnant women. Obstet Gynecol 2009;113:1285–91.

79. El Marroun H, Tiemeier H, Steegers EA, et al. Intrauterine cannabis exposure affects fetal growth trajectories: the Generation R Study. J Am Acad Child Adolesc Psychiatry 2009;48:1173–81.

80. Gouin K, Murphy K, Shah PS. Effects of cocaine use during pregnancy on low birthweight and preterm birth: systematic review and metaanalyses. Am J Obstet Gynecol 2011;204:340.e1–12.

81. Hulse GK, Milne E, English DR, et al. The relationship between maternal use of heroin and methadone and infant birth weight. Addiction 1997;92:1571–9.

82. Lester BM, Tronick EZ, LaGasse L, et al. The maternal lifestyle study: effects of substance exposure during pregnancy on neurodevelopmental outcome in 1-month-old infants. Pediatrics 2002;110:1182–92.

83. Goldschmidt L, Richardson GA, Cornelius MD, et al. Prenatal marijuana and alcohol exposure and academic achievement at age 10. Neurotoxicol Teratol 2004;26:521–32.

84. Patrick SW, Schumacher RE, Benneyworth BD, et al. Neonatal abstinence syndrome and associated health care expenditures: United States, 2000-2009. JAMA 2012;307:1934–40.

85. Frank DA, Jacobs RR, Beeghly M, et al. Level of prenatal cocaine exposure and scores on the Bayley Scales of Infant Development: modifying effects of caregiver, early intervention, and birth weight. Pediatrics 2002;110:1143–52.

86. Lumeng JC, Cabral HJ, Gannon K, et al. Pre-natal exposures to cocaine and alcohol and physical growth patterns to age 8 years. Neurotoxicol Teratol 2007;29:446–57.

87. Ingersoll KS, Ceperich SD, Hettema JE, et al. Preconceptional motivational interviewing interventions to reduce alcohol-exposed pregnancy risk. J Subst Abuse Treat 2013;44:407–16.

88. Humeniuk R, Ali R, Babor T, et al. A randomized controlled trial of a brief intervention for illicit drugs linked to the Alcohol, Smoking and Substance Involvement Screening Test (ASSIST) in clients recruited from primary health-care settings in four countries. Addiction 2012;107:957–66.

89. Terplan M, McNamara EJ, Chisolm MS. Pregnant and non-pregnant women with substance use disorders: The gap between treatment need and receipt. J Addict Dis 2012;31:342–9.

90. Greenfield SF, Brooks AJ, Gordon SM, et al. Substance abuse treatment entry, retention, and outcome in women: a review of the literature. Drug Alcohol Depend 2007;86:1–21.

91. Greenfield SF, Pettinati HM, O'Malley S, et al. Gender differences in alcohol treatment: an analysis of outcome from the COMBINE study. Alcohol Clin Exp Res 2010;34:1803–12.

92. Blume AW, Resor MR. Knowledge about health risks and drinking behavior among Hispanic women who are or have been of childbearing age. Addict Behav 2007;32:2335–9.

93. Tombor I, Urban R, Berkes T, et al. Denial of smoking-related risk among pregnant smokers. Acta Obstet Gynecol Scand 2010;89:524–30.

94. Binder T, Vavrinkova B. Prospective randomised comparative study of the effect of buprenorphine, methadone and heroin on the course of pregnancy, birthweight of newborns, early postpartum adaptation and course of the neonatal abstinence syndrome (NAS) in women followed up in the outpatient department. Neuro Endocrinol Lett 2008;29:80–6.

95. Burns L, Mattick RP, Lim K, et al. Methadone in pregnancy: treatment retention and neonatal outcomes. Addiction 2007;102:264–70.

96. Fajemirokun-Odudeyi O, Sinha C, Tutty S, et al. Pregnancy outcome in women who use opiates. Eur J Obstet Gynecol Reprod Biol 2006;126:170–5.

97. Jones HE, Kaltenbach K, Heil SH, et al. Neonatal abstinence syndrome after methadone or buprenorphine exposure. N Engl J Med 2010;363:2320–31.

98. Centers for Disease Control and Prevention. Frequently asked questions: alcohol and public health. 2013. Available at: http://www.cdc.gov/alcohol/faqs.htm. Accessed January 27, 2013.

99. National Institute on Alcohol Abuse and Alcoholism. Moderate & binge drinking. Available at: http://www.niaaa.nih.gov/alcohol-health/overview-alcohol-consumption/moderate-binge-drinking. Accessed January 27, 2013.

100. American Psychiatric Association. Diagnostic and statistical manual of mental disorders. 4th edition, text revision. Washington, DC: Author; 2000.

101. American Psychiatric Association. Diagnostic and statistical manual of mental disorders. 5th edition. Arlington (VA): American Psychiatric Publishing; 2013.

Adolescent Substance Use and Unplanned Pregnancy
Strategies for Risk Reduction

Hilary Smith Connery, MD, PhD[a,b,]*, Brittany B. Albright, MD, MPH[c],
John M. Rodolico, PhD[d,e]

KEYWORDS

- Adolescents • Substance use • Unintended pregnancy • Contraception
- Motivational interviewing

KEY POINTS

- Unplanned pregnancy is a significant public health issue, with rates being highest among adolescents. A main risk factor for unplanned pregnancy is alcohol and drug use.
- Adolescents are poorly trained to anticipate and recognize unplanned pregnancy. Fetal exposure to substances and late prenatal care may occur for many continuing to childbirth.
- It is recommended that primary care clinicians, including pediatricians and obstetrician-gynecologists, routinely screen adolescent patients for substance use.
- It is recommended that substance abuse treatment centers incorporate contraception and family planning education into their comprehensive treatment programs.
- Motivational interviewing effectively engages substance-using adolescents in treatments to reduce substance use and may also enhance pregnancy prevention in high-risk youths.

INTRODUCTION

Most US teen pregnancies are unplanned with preconception substance use being a significant risk factor for unintented pregnancy.[1] Both teenage pregnancy and teenage substance use are national public health concerns targeted for improved outcomes.[2] Unplanned pregnancies are associated with higher rates of maternal

Funding: NIH, U10DA15831; NIHMS-ID, 567747.
[a] Division of Alcohol and Drug Abuse, McLean Hospital, 115 Mill Street, Belmont, MA 02478, USA; [b] Department of Psychiatry, Harvard Medical School, Boston, MA, USA; [c] Massachusetts General Hospital/McLean Hospital Adult Psychiatry Residency Program, 15 Parkman Street, Wang 812, Boston, MA 02114, USA; [d] Division of Child and Adolescent Psychiatry, McLean Hospital, 115 Mill Street, Belmont, MA 02478, USA; [e] Clinical Psychology, Harvard Medical School, Boston, MA, USA
* Corresponding author. Division of Alcohol and Drug Abuse, McLean Hospital, 115 Mill Street, Mailstop 222, Belmont, MA 02478.
E-mail address: hconnery@mclean.harvard.edu

infections, obstetric complications, low birth weight, childhood growth stunting, poor child development, and subsequent child abuse or neglect.[3–6] Teen pregnancy and childbearing also have substantial economic and social costs: US taxpayers paid $10.9 billion in 2008 for costs associated with teen pregnancy, including increased health care, foster care, lost tax revenue, and higher incarceration rates among children of teen parents.[7]

This article presents recent data relevant to adolescent sexuality and substance use with the aim of defining strategies to reduce the risk of unplanned pregnancy in substance-using teens and to thereby protect healthy adolescent development and prevent fetal exposure to substances.

ADOLESCENT SUBSTANCE USE AND SEXUAL ACTIVITY

Teen substance use is an enduring problem in the United States. In 2011, 75% of high school students reported having used addictive substances, including tobacco, alcohol, marijuana, and other illicit drugs. Forty-six percent reported current use of addictive substances, and 1 in 3 substance-using students met the medical criteria for addiction.[8] According to the Monitoring the Future database survey results for 2012,[9] high school seniors self-report the following past-year substance use rates:

- 24% are binge drinkers (drank 5 or more drinks in a row at least once in the past 2 weeks)
- 17% are current tobacco cigarette smokers
- 8% misuse prescription opioids
- 6.5% are daily or near-daily marijuana users

These national data are consistent with other 2012 data showing 1 in 5 high school girls binge drink (defined as 4 or more drinks over 3 hours[10]).

Almost half (47.4%) of high school students have had sexual intercourse, and 22% of sexually active high school students reported having used alcohol or other drugs before their last sexual experience (26% of boys and 18% of girls).[11] Risk reduction efforts targeting safer sexual behavior is most relevant in teens who are 15 years of age and older because rates of sexual activity in the youngest adolescents (aged 10–14 years) are much lower than in adolescents aged 15 years and older; in those aged 12 years and younger, sexual activity is mostly nonconsensual, representing a different public health concern beyond the scope of this article (ie, preventing the sexual abuse of minors).[12]

UNPLANNED PREGNANCY AND SUBSTANCE USE

Defined by Finer and Zolna[1] (2013) as mistimed (pregnancy occurring sooner than desired) or unwanted pregnancies, unintended pregnancies are associated with potential health risks to the fetus because of delayed pregnancy recognition, with 58% of unplanned pregnancies being confirmed after 5 weeks' gestation.[5] More than half (51%) of all pregnancies in the United States in 2008 were unintended (rate of 54 unintended pregnancies per 1000 women aged 15–44 years), with 91% of all pregnancies in 15 to 17 year olds being unintended. Between 2001 and 2008, the rate increased for both unintended pregnancy and for those continuing an unplanned pregnancy to childbirth.[1] Therefore, delayed pregnancy recognition is more likely to result in inadequate prenatal care and unintentional fetal exposure to substances.

Rates of unintended pregnancies are higher among substance-using women, especially opioid users. Among treatment-seeking pregnant women with opioid-use disorders, 86% of pregnancies were reported to be unplanned.[13] Prospective self-report surveys of outpatient women in an Australian opioid treatment program revealed that nearly half (47%) had a teenage pregnancy and 84% of these were unplanned; nearly one-third of the sample were pregnant in the year before entry, with 75% of these pregnancies unplanned.[14] Risk factors associated with unplanned pregnancy included substance intoxication during sexual activity and lack of contraceptive use.

Among white women participating in a large national community sample study using case control methods (N = 72,907; Pregnancy Risk Assessment Monitoring System), preconception binge drinking was significantly associated with unplanned pregnancy and was also predictive of alcohol and tobacco use during pregnancy.[5]

The relationships among age, substance use, and risky sexual behavior for unplanned pregnancy are complex and frequently confounded by other high-risk demographic factors, such as race/ethnicity, poverty, lower education, being a victim of abuse, being the child of a teenage mother, co-occurring mental illness, and lack of access to health care.[15–17] Adolescents who are sexually active and use substances have high rates of unintended pregnancy and of repeat unplanned pregnancy for multiple reasons. Teens that use tobacco, alcohol, marijuana, or other drugs are more likely to be sexually active; to engage in risky sexual behavior; and to experience the consequences of risky sex, including unintended pregnancy, compared with peers who do not use substances.[8] Moreover, a sexually active teen has high fertility; for teens aged 16 to 19 years, the probability of becoming pregnant is 2 to 5 times more likely for teens not using contraception at first sexual intercourse compared with those who did use contraception at first sexual intercourse.[17] The more forms of addictive substances a teen uses in his or her lifetime, the less likely that teen is to report condom use at last intercourse.[8,18] Absence of any teen contraceptive use is high: half of pregnant teens aged 15 to 18 years were not using contraception when they became pregnant, and 31% of these thought they could not get pregnant at the time.[11]

PREGNANT TEEN SUBSTANCE USE

The most recent national estimates of substance use among pregnant teenagers are known from self-report data in the large National Survey on Drug Use and Health.[10] In the 2011–2012 pooled data for pregnant teens aged 15 to 17 years, 18.3% reported past-month illicit drug use, a significant increase from 2009 to 2010 (15.7%). Young pregnant teens reported greater drug use compared with same-age nonpregnant peers (13.8%), double the rate of pregnant youth aged 18 to 25 years (9%), and 6 times the rate of pregnant women aged 26 to 44 years (3.4%). The specific drugs used remains stable, with marijuana, cocaine, and prescription medications (mainly opioid analgesics) being the top 3 reported in order of greatest frequency of use among all pregnant women aged 15 to 44 years.

Past-month alcohol use is significantly less among pregnant youth aged 18 to 25 years compared with age-matched nonpregnant peers (7% vs 60%). In contrast, pregnant teens aged 15 to 17 years are drinking at half the rate of age-matched nonpregnant peers (13.4% vs 21.6%) and double the rate of pregnant youths. These rates are unchanged since 2009 to 2010.

Past-month cigarette use is unknown for adolescents aged 15 to 17 years but nearly 21% for adolescents aged 18 to 25 years. Although data for all pregnant women aged 15 to 44 years indicate that rates of second- and third-trimester use of alcohol and drugs decreased to less than 5%, tobacco use persists at rates of 13.6% and 11.1% in second and third trimester, respectively. These data are alarming given the teratogenic effects of prenatal exposure to addictive substances reviewed by Connery and Rayburn in this issue and previously by Behnke and Smith.[19] Furthermore, these estimates may underrepresent true rates of fetal exposure because of the reluctance to disclose substance use, especially among underaged users and pregnant women.

SCREENING ADOLESCENTS FOR SUBSTANCE USE

Although many evidence-based office tools exist to assist clinicians in screening for substance use (reviewed in Refs.[20,21]), including brief screens such as the T-ACE[22] and TWEAK[23] for use in pregnant women, among assessments the authors recommend the use of the CRAFFT screening tool, which was designed specifically for use in adolescents and has been validated in multiple community- and hospital-based clinical contexts.[24–27] It has also been effectively used to detect preconception substance use in a small cohort of pregnant women aged 17 to 25 years.[28] **Fig. 1** outlines instructions, question item content, and scoring for the CRAFFT.

The CRAFFT Screening Interview

Begin: "I'm going to ask you a few questions that I ask all my patients. Please be honest. I will keep your answers confidential."

Part A

During the PAST 12 MONTHS, did you: No   Yes

1. Drink any <u>alcohol</u> (more than a few sips)?   ☐   ☐
(Do not count sips of alcohol taken during family or religious events.)

2. Smoke any <u>marijuana or hashish</u>?   ☐   ☐

3. Use <u>anything else</u> to <u>get high</u>?   ☐   ☐
("anything else" includes illegal drugs, over the counter and
prescription drugs, and things that you sniff or "huff")

For clinic use only: Did the patient answer "yes" to any questions in Part A?

No ☐   Yes ☐

↓   ↓

Ask CAR question only, then stop   **Ask all 6 CRAFFT questions**

Part B   No   Yes

1. Have you ever ridden in a **CAR** driven by someone (including yourself) who   ☐   ☐
was "high" or had been using alcohol or drugs?

2. Do you ever use alcohol or drugs to **RELAX**, feel better about yourself, or fit   ☐   ☐
in?

3. Do you ever use alcohol or drugs while you are by yourself, or **ALONE**?   ☐   ☐

4. Do you ever **FORGET** things you did while using alcohol or drugs?   ☐   ☐

5. Do your **FAMILY** or **FRIENDS** ever tell you that you should cut down on your   ☐   ☐
drinking or drug use?

6. Have you ever gotten into **TROUBLE** while you were using alcohol or drugs?   ☐   ☐

Fig. 1. The CRAFFT Screening Interview.

SCORING INSTRUCTIONS: FOR CLINIC STAFF USE ONLY

CRAFFT Scoring: Each "yes" response in **Part B** scores 1 point.
A total score of 2 or higher is a positive screen, indicating a need for additional assessment.

Probability of Substance Abuse/Dependence Diagnosis Based on CRAFFT Score[1,2]

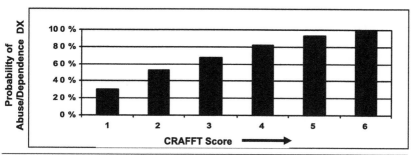

DSM-IV Diagnostic Criteria[3] (Abbreviated)

Substance Abuse (1 or more of the following):
- Use causes failure to fulfill obligations at work, school, or home
- Recurrent use in hazardous situations (e.g. driving)
- Recurrent legal problems
- Continued use despite recurrent problems

Substance Dependence (3 or more of the following):
- Tolerance
- Withdrawal
- Substance taken in larger amount or over longer period of time than planned
- Unsuccessful efforts to cut down or quit
- Great deal of time spent to obtain substance or recover from effect
- Important activities given up because of substance
- Continued use despite harmful consequences

© Children's Hospital Boston, 2009. This form may be reproduced in its exact form for use in clinical settings, courtesy of the Center for Adolescent Substance Abuse Research, Children's Hospital Boston, 300 Longwood Ave, Boston, MA 02115, U.S.A., (617) 355-5433, www.ceasar.org.

References:
1. Knight JR, Shrier LA, Bravender TD, Farrell M, Vander Bilt J, Shaffer HJ. A new brief screen for adolescent substance abuse. Arch Pediatr Adolesc Med 1999;153(6):591-6.
2. Knight JR, Sherritt L, Shrier LA, Harris SK, Chang G. Validity of the CRAFFT substance abuse screening test among adolescent clinic patients. Arch Pediatr Adolesc Med 2002;156(6):607-14.
3. American Psychiatric Association. Diagnostic and Statistical Manual of Mental Disorders, fourth edition, text revision. Washington DC, American Psychiatric Association, 2000.

Fig. 1. (*continued*)

Advantages of the CRAFFT

The CRAFFT has several advantages:

- Free public access
- No training required
- 2 to 3 minutes to complete
- Screens both alcohol and drug use simultaneously, with good positive and negative predictive probability for problem use, abuse, and dependence
- 74% sensitivity and 96% specificity

- Computerized version validated and can be incorporated into other screening programs[29]
- Available in many languages

Limitations of the CRAFFT

Limitations of the CRAFFT include

- Not a comprehensive assessment of substance use
- Needs a separate screen for tobacco products, e-cigarettes, and hookah vaping; typically single-item questions about ever-use followed by quantification for positive screens[30–33]
- Requires knowledgeable interpretation for risk assessment
- Not intended to measure treatment outcomes

Positive screens on the CRAFFT provide an opportunity for follow-up conversations regarding substance use health risks, including risky sexual behavior and unplanned pregnancy. Separate screening for nicotine use is also recommended, especially as teenage cigarette smoking is associated with higher rates of co-occurring mental illness and substance abuse.[30] Although brief educational follow-up may be helpful, educational content delivered within the context of a motivational enhancement session is likely to have more impact.

MOTIVATIONAL INTERVIEWING IN ADOLESCENTS
What is Motivational Interviewing?

Motivational interviewing (MI) is a client-centered, collaborative approach to eliciting and strengthening motivation for change and evoking ideas and plans for changing behavior.[34] MI is well suited to working with clients who are difficult to engage in treatment (eg, adolescents, substance users, and those with high-risk lifestyles) because it always engages clients from their position of autonomy and resourcefulness. The interventionist's primary tasks are twofold: first, to recognize and verbally reinforce "change talk" (statements oriented toward desire, ability, reason, or need to change behavior) using empathic reflections that highlight change talk while ignoring other verbalizations associated with barriers to change or "sustain talk" (commonly called *resistance* to change) and, second, to assist clients in formulating plans, actions, and commitments to change drawing on the clients' inherent resourcefulness and adding collaborative expertise and strategy when this is sought by clients. MI has a very strong evidence base for promoting change and is popular with clinicians because its spirit is compassionate and its emphasis on client responsibility reduces frustration and burnout. MI does require training and practice to learn, and many opportunities for clinician training are provided through the MI Network of Trainers (www.motivationalinterviewing.org).

Does MI Reduce Substance Use in Adolescents?

There is ample evidence of MI's efficacy in reducing teen substance use. Barnett and colleagues[35] (2012) reviewed the literature and cited 26 clinical trials of good quality, with participants younger than 18 years showing at least modest effects on improving substance use outcomes, including alcohol, tobacco, and marijuana, the 3 most commonly used substances among preconception and pregnant teens. The number of MI sessions delivered ranged from 1 to more than 3, and studies that included personalized feedback were no more effective than studies that did not include a feedback component. Individual MI sessions composed the most studies, and the efficacy of MI in a group-treatment setting remains uncertain. When feedback was provided, in-person feedback was superior to computerized feedback, but in-person sessions did not seem to always be superior to telephone sessions. Involving parents as part of the delivered interventions (for instance, adding a component of addiction education for the parent) seems to support improved outcomes. More suggestive evidence is provided by a Cochrane review of 28 clinical trials targeting adolescent smoking cessation.[31] The researchers concluded that, although current evidence does not yet support clear recommendations, the most promising studies (ie, those demonstrating postintervention abstinence at 30 days or 6 months continuous abstinence) incorporated an MI or motivational enhancement intervention.

MI is a natural match for engaging adolescents because they are focused on developing autonomy and discovering their own capacities. When clinicians are adherent to the spirit of MI, adolescents are more welcoming of conversations related to risk reduction, self-efficacy development, and collaborative goal setting. Practical applications and adaptations for adolescent treatment, including articles on substance use and risky sexual behavior, are well outlined in Naar-King and Suarez's[36] textbook (2011).

Can MI Reduce Risk of Unplanned Teen Pregnancy?

Only one randomized controlled clinical trial using computer-assisted MI as part of a home- and community-delivered intervention to prevent repeat pregnancy, conducted in a population of at-risk African American adolescents, informs us about the potential benefit of MI in teens at high risk for unplanned pregnancy.[37] Paraprofessionals selected for their empathy and knowledge of participant culture and norms received 2.5 days of training and certification as MI interventionists followed by 4 months fidelity monitoring and feedback using audiotaped sessions. The MI intervention consisted of computer self-report on sexual behaviors and contraceptive use, and data resulted in assessment of contraceptive use stage of change and feedback on risk for pregnancy. The MI interventionists then conducted a 20-minute stage-matched MI session to enhance motivation for contraceptive use and avoiding pregnancy. At least 7 sessions had to be delivered, the first within 6 weeks post partum, in order to count as a completed intervention. The results showed MI alone did not significantly reduce 24-month repeat pregnancy, whereas MI plus parent training/case management (MI+) intervention significantly reduced pregnancy rates compared with office-based treatment as usual ($P<.05$). It is noted that the MI+ group was more adherent than the MI-alone group, with sooner transition of phone contact to in-home visits; this may have affected outcomes.

Among adult women at risk for unplanned pregnancy because of risky drinking and high-risk for ineffective contraceptive use, 2 brief counseling interventions using MI plus personalized feedback, CHOICES (delivered as four 30- to 75-minute sessions) and BALANCE (an adaptation of CHOICES for a college sample of youths aged 18–25 years, delivered as one 60-minute session), coupled with a medical contraception counseling appointment (in BALANCE, this was strongly encouraged but not delivered with the intervention) have been tested in randomized controlled trials.[38–41] Interventions in both studies were compared with an informational brochure to reduce the risk of unplanned pregnancy by reviewing topics of fetal alcohol spectrum disorder, women's health and contraception, and mental health and substance use. Both of these MI-based interventions were superior to control for reducing risky drinking, improving contraception rates, and decreasing absolute risk of alcohol-exposed pregnancies (absolute risk reduction in CHOICES was 18% and BALANCE was 15%).

As a follow-up, in an effort to adapt these treatments to better serve real-world practice and community samples, the researchers examined the effect of one 60-minute

MI session plus assessment feedback (EARLY) in a community sample of women at risk for unplanned pregnancy because of risky drinking and ineffective contraceptive behavior.[42] Informational videos (45 minutes) or a brochure on relevant topic content were the two control comparisons. All interventions showed statistically significant, modest reductions in drinks per drinking day, ineffective contraception rates, and alcohol-exposed pregnancies over a 3-month period; EARLY was superior to the informational controls in reducing alcohol-exposed pregnancies at 3 months (absolute risk reduction 6.3% vs video and 8.3% vs brochure). Although the effects were smaller in magnitude when compared with multisession CHOICES, this intervention provides an effective alternative when a more intensive intervention is not feasible. It should be noted that MI interventionists in this study had either master's or doctoral level training, completed extensive prestudy MI training and certification, and participated in weekly MI supervision including review of audiotaped sessions to ensure protocol adherence and fidelity to MI intervention. This aspect of the study as it pertains to successful outcomes must not be overlooked when clinical settings are considering applications of this type of intervention; the need for high-quality training and longitudinal supervision in motivational interventions is a well-documented determinant of intervention efficacy.[43]

SUBSTANCE ABUSE TREATMENT PROGRAMS: ROLE IN REDUCING RISK FOR UNPLANNED PREGNANCY
Need for Family Planning Services in Substance Abuse Treatment Programs

Women account for approximately 30% to 40% of patients attending substance use treatment programs, yet these programs do not routinely address women's reproductive health.[44] By integrating reproductive services into substance abuse treatment, patients have improved maternal health through facilitated access in a less threatening environment.[45]

Specific guidelines and policies are lacking in substance abuse treatment centers for family planning. Perhaps this is because of the fact that family planning implies intentional consideration of becoming (or not becoming) a mother, and women presenting to general substance use treatment centers are often in crisis and commonly suffering the acute symptoms of co-occurring mental illness, such as suicidal ideation, psychosis, severe anxiety, and trauma-related disorders. Quality treatment typically includes screening for risky sexual behaviors and strategies to reduce such exposures in order to avoid sexually transmitted diseases, becoming a victim of physical or sexual abuse, and unintended pregnancy. Although health care referral options are made available if a woman discovers she is pregnant while in treatment, specific contraceptive counseling and family planning interventions are often absent or inadequately addressed, being deferred to the next referral point of care. Routine brief interventions focus on the health of the woman in treatment and may avoid discussion of the unintended effects of drugs and alcohol on her baby should she become pregnant and the impact of this on her own psychological health in the future. Because data suggest that substance-using pregnant teens and women effectively reduce alcohol and drug use in second and third trimesters, it may be that current treatment practice underestimates this valued incentive to change among most substance-using women entering treatment programs. Additionally, the lack of equivalent reduction rates of tobacco use in later pregnancy may well reflect another problem needing to be addressed in substance abuse treatment: the need to correct clinician and client perceptions about tobacco use as a lethal drug use disorder and to provide relevant access to care and reimbursement schedules for evidence-based tobacco cessation treatments.[46]

Pregnancy Diagnosed in the Context of Substance Abuse Treatment

Women and teens with active substance use diagnosed with an unplanned pregnancy should be referred to an obstetrician for prenatal care and more intensive substance abuse counseling if patients elect to continue their pregnancy. Comprehensive referrals are needed to adequately address the mental health risks of pregnant and parenting teen mothers, particularly high rates of depression (16%–44%), stress and trauma-related disorders, and substance use.[47]

Approximately half of unintended pregnancies in the United States are terminated by elective abortion[48]; studies report that resolution of an unintended pregnancy by induced abortion is associated with higher maternal rates of alcohol consumption, nicotine dependence, and illegal drug use.[49,50] Elective abortion among adolescents seems to be medically safe,[51,52] but there are little data to guide clinicians on appropriate mental health monitoring after abortion. Aftercare planning is, therefore, typically determined by client history and the presenting risk factors. Conservative decision making on monitoring frequency and anticipation of possible delayed mental health symptoms is warranted.

COMMON OPPORTUNITIES TO REDUCE UNPLANNED TEEN PREGNANCY

According to the Centers for Disease Control and Prevention's (CDC) 2011 surveys, only 65% of teenaged girls and 53% of teenaged boys received formal sex education about both abstinence and birth control, and only 44% of teenaged girls and 27% of teenaged boys report having talked with their parents about abstinence and birth control. Clinicians may use MI styles and strategies to effectively engage teens in conversations about sensitive topical content in order to optimally educate clients and to promote and support self-efficacy for behavioral risk reduction. These topics also provide opportunistic targets, with teen permission, for engaging family and friends in active support of healthy choices and behaviors. **Box 1** outlines recommended brief interventions consistent with MI principles and practices that, based on the current evidence, we would consider "best practices" for reducing risk related to teen substance use, sexual behavior, and unintended pregnancy.

Box 1
Strategies to increase perceived risks of unplanned pregnancy and substance use

- Elicit and clarify teen's perceptions of risk and why these matter to him or her
- Positively reinforce correct perceptions
- Ask permission to review topics whereby risk perception is missing or inaccurate
- Use personalized examples based on elicited goals and values
- Complement brief conversations with multimedia/interactive exercises on risk assessment
- Evoke teen ideas and commitments to reducing risk behavior
- Encourage collaborative support from family and friends and invite ideas to involve them
- Follow up on commitments to establish continuity and support self-efficacy
- Refer to specialist adjuncts as indicated by severity of immediate risk

Data from Kirby D, Coyle K, Alton F, et al. Reducing adolescent sexual risk: a theoretical guide for developing and adapting curriculum-based programs. Scotts Valley (CA): ETR Associates; 2011; and Naar-King S, Suarez M. Motivational interviewing with adolescents and young adults. New York: Guilford Press; 2011.

The CDC recommends that health care providers increase the availability of birth control to sexually active teens and offer teens long-acting reversible birth control, such as intrauterine devices (IUDs) or long-acting implants.[53] Communities are asked to increase access to reproductive services and sex education that have been proven efficacious in preventing unintended pregnancy.

These recommendations are controversial with regard to religious and cultural freedoms and respect for the family of origin preferences/beliefs; thus, clinicians and communities experience important challenges in implementing interventions that would protect teens from unplanned pregnancy while remaining neutral and respectful of family and individual choices. MI, with its emphasis on autonomy, empathy, and clear comprehension of client goals and values, provides an evidence-supported tool for discussing sensitive public health recommendations while maintaining respect and professional neutrality.

For sexually active teens, barriers to optimal contraceptive use include access to health care providers, cost of contraception, concerns about confidentiality, negative attitudes about contraception, concerns about side effects, low self-efficacy, poor communication with partner, and partner resistance to contraception.[54] The most commonly used and least expensive forms of contraception, oral contraceptives and condoms, have high failure rates caused in large part by problems with adherence.[55,56] Substance use further impairs proper adherence because of intoxication at time of use, forgetfulness, and lack of structure in lifestyle. Reduction of substance use is here considered an important target for contraceptive adherence or, for those not using contraceptives, for supporting self-efficacy in abstinence or limiting sexual activity to safe, committed partners with whom family planning has been fully addressed.

Increased use of long-acting methods that minimize the risk of human error, such as the IUD and hormone implants, could play an important role in preventing pregnancy among substance users.[57] The American Congress of Obstetricians and Gynecologists indicated that such methods should be first-line choices for young women, and coupling IUDs with condoms for additional protection may have the potential to reduce unintended pregnancy even further.[58,59] One major barrier to using these longer-term methods is the up-front out-of-pocket cost for uninsured or underinsured women despite the fact that they are significantly cost-effective over time. Economic modeling of the costs of unintended pregnancy using a third-party payer database demonstrated that 53% of unintended pregnancies were caused by imperfect adherence with reversible contraceptive methods and that savings in the millions would be possible if even 10% of women in their twenties switched from oral contraceptives to longer-acting contraception.[60] As lower-income women have higher rates of unintended pregnancy resulting in childbirth,[1] providing financial access to health care options, including family planning and pregnancy prevention, substance use treatment when indicated, and prenatal care, are especially important in a population that is more difficult to engage in comprehensive health care.

REFERENCES

1. Finer LB, Zolna MR. Shifts in intended and unintended pregnancies in the United States, 2001–2008. Am J Public Health 2013. [Epub Ahead of Print]. http://dx.doi.org/10.2105/AJPH.2013.301416.
2. USHHS Healthy People 2020, Topics: adolescent health. Available at: http://www.healthypeople.gov/2020/topicsobjectives2020/overview.aspx?topicid=2. Accessed January 18, 2014.

3. Institute of Medicine. The best intentions: unintended pregnancy and the well-being of children and families. In: Brown SS, Eisenberg L, editors. Committee on Unintended Pregnancy, Division of Health Promotion and Disease Prevention. Washington, DC: National Academy Press; 1995. p. 202–3.
4. Baydar N. Consequences for children of their birth planning status. Fam Plann Perspect 1995;27:228–45.
5. Naimi TS, Lipscomb LE, Brewer RD, et al. Binge drinking in the preconception period and the risk of unintended pregnancy: implications for women and their children. Pediatrics 2003;111:1136.
6. Shapiro-Mendoza C, Selwyn BJ, Smith DP, et al. Parental pregnancy intention and early childhood stunting: findings from Bolivia. Int J Epidemiol 2005; 34(2):387–96.
7. National Campaign to Prevent Teen and Unplanned Pregnancy. Counting it up: the public costs of teen childbearing. 2011. Available at: http://www.thenational campaign.org/costs/default.aspx. Accessed December 22, 2013.
8. Adolescent substance use: America's #1 public health problem. The National Center on Addiction and Substance Abuse at Columbia University. 2011. Available at: http://www.casacolumbia.org/upload/2011/20110629adolescentsubstanceuse. pdf. Accessed December 22, 2013.
9. Johnston LD, O'Malley PM, Bachman JG, et al. Monitoring the future: national results on drug use: 2012 overview, key findings on adolescent drug use. Ann Arbor (MI): Institute for Social Research, The University of Michigan; 2013.
10. Substance Abuse and Mental Health Services Administration. Results from the 2012 National Survey on Drug Use and Health: Summary of National Findings, NSDUH Series H-46, HHS Publication No. (SMA) 13–4795. Rockville (MD): Substance Abuse and Mental Health Services Administration; 2013.
11. CDC. Youth risk behavior surveillance—United States, 2011. MMWR Surveill Summ 2012;61(SS-4):1–162.
12. Finer LB, Philbin JM. Sexual initiation, contraceptive use, and pregnancy among young adolescents. Pediatrics 2013;131(5):886–91.
13. Heil SH, Jones HE, Arria A, et al. Unintended pregnancy in opioid-abusing women. J Subst Abuse Treat 2011;40(2):199–202.
14. Black KI, Stephens C, Haber PS, et al. Unplanned pregnancy and contraceptive use in women attending drug treatment services. Aust N Z J Obstet Gynaecol 2012;52:146–50.
15. Kotchick BA, Shaffer A, Miller KS, et al. Adolescent sexual risk behavior: a multi-system perspective. Clin Psychol Rev 2001;21(4):493–519.
16. Meade CS, Ickovics JR. Systematic review of sexual risk among pregnant and mothering teens in the USA: pregnancy as an opportunity for integrated prevention of STD and repeat pregnancy. Soc Sci Med 2005;60(4):661–78.
17. Martinez G, Copen CE, Abma JC. Teenagers in the United States: sexual activity, contraceptive use, and childbearing, 2006–2010 National Survey of Family Growth. National Center for Health Statistics. Vital Health Stat 2011;23(31):1–35.
18. Santelli JS, Robin L, Brener ND, et al. Timing of alcohol and other drug use and sexual risk behaviors among unmarried adolescents and young adults. Fam Plann Perspect 2001;33(5):200–5.
19. Behnke M, Smith VC, Committee on Substance Abuse, Committee on Fetus and Newborn. Prenatal substance abuse: short- and long-term effects on the exposed fetus. Pediatrics 2013;131(3):e1009–24.
20. Burns E, Gray R, Smith LA. Brief screening questionnaires to identify problem drinking during pregnancy: a systematic review. Addiction 2010;105(4):601–14.

21. Goodman DJ, Wolff KB. Screening for substance abuse in women's health: a public health imperative. J Midwifery Womens Health 2013;58:278–87.
22. Sokol RJ, Martier SS, Ager JW. The T-ACE questions: practical prenatal detection of risk-drinking. Am J Obstet Gynecol 1989;160:863–8 [discussion: 868–70].
23. Russell M, Bigler L. Screening for alcohol-related problems in an outpatient obstetric–gynecologic clinic. Am J Obstet Gynecol 1979;134:4–12.
24. Knight JR, Shrier LA, Bravender TD, et al. A new brief screen for adolescent substance abuse. Arch Pediatr Adolesc Med 1999;153(6):591–6.
25. Knight JR, Sherritt L, Shrier LA, et al. Validity of the CRAFFT substance abuse screening test among adolescent clinic patients. Arch Pediatr Adolesc Med 2002;156:607–14.
26. Knight JR, Sherritt L, Harris SK, et al. Validity of the brief alcohol screening tests among adolescents: a comparison of the AUDIT, POSIT, CAGE, and CRAFFT. Alcohol Clin Exp Res 2003;27:67–73.
27. Dhalla S, Zumbo BD, Poole G. A review of the psychometric properties of the CRAFFT instrument: 1999-2010. Curr Drug Abuse Rev 2011;4(1):57–64.
28. Chang G, Orav EJ, Jones JA, et al. Self-reported alcohol and drug use in pregnant young women: a pilot study of associated factors and identification. J Addict Med 2011;5(3):221–6.
29. Knight JR, Harris SK, Sherritt L, et al. Adolescents' preference for substance abuse screening in primary care practice. J Subst Abuse Treat 2007;28(4):107–17.
30. Chang G, Sherritt L, Knight JR. Adolescent cigarette smoking and mental health symptoms. J Adolesc Health 2005;36(6):517–22.
31. Stanton A, Grimshaw G. Tobacco cessation interventions for young people. Cochrane Database Syst Rev 2013;(8):CD003289.
32. Palazzolo DL. Electronic cigarettes and vaping: a new challenge in clinical medicine and public health. A literature review. Front Public Health 2013;1:56.
33. Barnett TE, Forrest JR, Porter L, et al. A multiyear assessment of hookah use prevalence among Florida high school students. Nicotine Tob Res 2014;16(3):373–7.
34. Miller WR, Rollnick S. Motivational interviewing (3rd edition): helping people change. New York: Guilford Press; 2012.
35. Barnett E, Sussman S, Smith C, et al. Motivational Interviewing for adolescent substance use: a review of the literature. Addict Behav 2012;37(12):1325–34.
36. Naar-King S, Suarez M. Motivational interviewing with adolescents and young adults. New York: Guilford Press; 2011.
37. Barnet B, Liu J, DeVoe M, et al. Motivational intervention to reduce rapid subsequent births to adolescent mothers: community-based randomized trial. Ann Fam Med 2009;7(5):436–45.
38. Ingersoll K, Floyd L, Sobell M, et al, Project CHOICES Intervention Research Group. Reducing the risk of alcohol-exposed pregnancies: a study of a motivational intervention in community settings. Pediatrics 2003;111:1131–5.
39. Ingersoll KS, Ceperich SD, Nettleman MD, et al. Reducing alcohol-exposed pregnancy risk in college women: initial outcomes of a clinical trial of a motivational intervention. J Subst Abuse Treat 2005;29:173–80.
40. Floyd RL, Sobell M, Velasquez MM, et al. Preventing alcohol-exposed pregnancies: a randomized controlled trial. Am J Prev Med 2007;32:1–10.
41. Ceperich SD, Ingersoll KS. Motivational interviewing + feedback intervention to reduce alcohol-exposed pregnancy risk among college binge drinkers: determinants and patterns of response. J Behav Med 2011;34:381–95.

42. Ingersoll KS, Ceperich SD, Hettema JE, et al. Preconception motivational interviewing interventions to reduce alcohol-exposed pregnancy risk. J Subst Abuse Treat 2013;44(4):407–16.
43. Martino S, Ball SA, Nich C, et al. Community program therapist adherence and competence in motivational enhancement therapy. Drug Alcohol Depend 2008; 96(1–2):37–48.
44. Sherman SG, Kamarulzaman A, Spittal P. Women and drugs across the globe: a call to action. Int J Drug Policy 2008;19(2):97–8.
45. Niccols A, Milligan K, Sword W, et al. Maternal mental health and integrated programs for mothers with substance abuse issues. Psychol Addict Behav 2010; 24:466–74.
46. Williams JM, Willett JG, Miller G. Partnership between tobacco control programs and offices of mental health needed to reduce smoking rates in the United States. JAMA Psychiatry 2013;70(12):1261–2.
47. Hodgkinson S, Beers L, Southammakosane C, et al. Addressing the mental health needs of pregnant and parenting adolescents. Pediatrics 2014;133(1): 114–22.
48. Finer LB, Henshaw SK. Disparities in rates of unintended pregnancy in the United States, 1994 and 2001. Perspect Sex Reprod Health 2006;38(2):90–6.
49. Reardon DC, Coleman PK, Cougle JR. Substance use associated with unintended pregnancy outcomes in the national longitudinal survey of youth. Am J Drug Alcohol Abuse 2004;30(2):369–83.
50. Pedersen W. Childbirth, abortion and subsequent substance use in young women: a population-based longitudinal study. Addiction 2007;102(12):1971–8.
51. Renner RM, de Guzman A, Brahmi D. Abortion care for adolescent and young women. Int J Gynaecol Obstet 2013. [Epub ahead of print].
52. Kirby D, Coyle K, Alton F, et al. Reducing adolescent sexual risk: a theoretical guide for developing and adapting curriculum-based programs. Scotts Valley (CA): ETR Associates; 2011. Available at: http://pub.etr.org/upfiles/Reducing_Adolescent_Sexual_Risk.pdf.
53. CDC Vital Signs. Preventing teen pregnancy in the US. Centers for Disease Control; 2011. Available at: http://www.cdc.gov/VitalSigns/pdf/2011-04-vitalsigns.pdf. Accessed October 5, 2013.
54. Coles MS, Makino KK, Stanwood NL. Contraceptive experiences among adolescents who experience unintended birth. Contraception 2011;84(6):578–84.
55. Trussell J, Wynn LL. Reducing unintended pregnancy in the United States. Contraception 2008;77:1–5.
56. Blumenthal PD, Voedisch A, Gemzell-Danielsson K. Strategies to prevent unintended pregnancy: increasing use of long-acting reversible contraception. Hum Reprod Update 2011;17:121–37.
57. Winner B, Peipert JF, Zhao Q, et al. Effectiveness of long-acting reversible contraception. N Engl J Med 2012;366:1998–2007.
58. ACOG Committee on Practice Bulletins. Clinical management guidelines for obstetrician-gynecologists: intrauterine device. Obstet Gynecol 2005;105: 223–32.
59. Finer LB, Zolna MR. Unintended pregnancy in the United States: incidence and disparities, 2006. Contraception 2011;84(5):478–85.
60. Trussell J, Henry N, Hassan F, et al. Burden of unintended pregnancy in the United States: potential savings with increased use of long-acting reversible contraception. Contraception 2013;87(2):154–61.

Screening for Alcohol and Drug Use During Pregnancy

Grace Chang, MD, MPH[a,b,*]

KEYWORDS

- Biomarkers • Questionnaires • Sensitivity • Specificity

KEY POINTS

- The use of alcohol and other substances is not infrequent during pregnancy but may not be routinely disclosed by women.
- Screening all pregnant women for their use of substances with an approach that is suited to the clinical setting has been recommended.
- A positive screen is not a diagnosis, but an opportunity for the clinician and patient to review health practices, and to make necessary changes.

INTRODUCTION

The 2012 National Survey on Drug Use and Health showed that among pregnant women in the past month, approximately 5.9% had used substances, 8.5% had consumed alcohol, and 15.9% smoked cigarettes.[1] A five-fold increase in antepartum maternal opioid use coincident with an "epidemic" of opioid prescription abuse between 2000 and 2009 has also been reported, with young women being as likely as men to abuse opioid medications.[2,3] Among women of childbearing age, one-fifth between the ages of 15 and 17 used illicit substances in the past month.[1] Moreover, the gender gap in alcohol use, abuse, and dependence in the United States is closing among women of childbearing age, so that the rates of alcohol consumption by women are approaching those of men.[4] Indeed, the estimate of past month alcohol use is potentially misleading, because 30.3% of nearly 4100 pregnant women who delivered a live-born infant without birth defects acknowledged that they drank alcohol while pregnant.[5]

Adverse consequences may be associated with prenatal exposure to any of these substances. Many pregnant women continue to smoke cigarettes, drink alcohol, or use other substances throughout pregnancy and after delivery, unless these practices

[a] Harvard Medical School, 25 Shattuck Street, Boston, MA 02115, USA; [b] Department of Psychiatry, VA Boston Healthcare System, 940 Belmont Street, Brockton, MA 02301, USA
* Department of Psychiatry, VA Boston Healthcare System, 940 Belmont Street, Brockton, MA 02301.
E-mail address: Grace.Chang2@va.gov

Obstet Gynecol Clin N Am 41 (2014) 205–212
http://dx.doi.org/10.1016/j.ogc.2014.02.002
0889-8545/14/$ – see front matter Published by Elsevier Inc.

obgyn.theclinics.com

are recognized and addressed. Hence, it is desirable to facilitate identification early in pregnancy to optimize outcomes for all.

Screening may be one way to achieve consistent and early identification. Methods of screening include the use of questionnaires or biomarkers. Complicated ethical issues have been described to be associated with screening for biomarkers of prenatal alcohol exposure. Such ethical concerns include selecting which patients are screened, their potential stigmatization, accuracy of testing, confidentiality, appropriate follow-up to positive screen results, and the use of screening results for criminal prosecution.[6] These concerns could be applicable to any type of screening for other substances used in the antepartum.

After careful consideration of the principles of beneficence, nonmaleficence, justice, and respect for autonomy, the Committee on Ethics from the American College of Obstetricians and Gynecologists expressed its support of universal screening questions, brief intervention, and referral to treatment: "obstetrician-gynecologists have an ethical obligation to learn and use a protocol for universal screening questions, brief intervention, and referral to treatment, in order to provide patients and their families with medical care that is state-of-the art, comprehensive, and effective."[7]

SCREENING OPTIONS

The identification of prenatal alcohol and other substance use is challenging. Health care professionals may be reticent to inquire about these practices and patients may be reluctant to disclose them because of stigma, denial, or change in behavior after pregnancy confirmation. Fears about legal and other sanctions may also contribute to nondisclosure.[6,8,9] Finally, whereas the development and evaluation of screening measures for prenatal alcohol use is well advanced, the validity, reliability, and clinical use of standardized questionnaires in screening for illicit drug use during pregnancy is not commensurate.[10,11]

Indeed, the US Preventive Services Task Force has issued several recommendations with regards to tobacco and alcohol use by adult women. It has issued a Grade A recommendation that clinicians ask all pregnant women about tobacco use and provide augmented, pregnancy-tailored counseling for those who smoke.[12] Similarly, it has issued a Grade B recommendation that clinicians screen for alcohol misuse by adults (including pregnant women) and provide brief behavioral counseling interventions; moreover, complete abstinence is recommended for pregnant women.[13] However, the US Preventive Services Task Force has concluded that there is insufficient evidence to evaluate the benefits and harms of screening for illicit drug use in clinical populations including pregnant women because the validity, reliability, and clinical use of standardized questionnaires in screening for illicit drug use during pregnancy have not been adequately evaluated.[11]

Biomarkers

Biomarkers of alcohol and drug exposure have been considered as one approach to the identification of prenatal alcohol or drug use. Toxicologic tests of blood or urine have been used in other settings to provide objective evidence of drug use in many settings. However, such tests do not distinguish between occasional users and those who use more regularly.[11] In addition, the short half-life of some substances limits detection only to recent use. For example, ethanol and acetaldehyde are measured for a few hours after ethanol intake in conventional matrices, such as blood, urine, and sweat.[14] Similar limitations apply to urine or saliva screens for use of cocaine and heroin, so that positive results only reflect very recent use within the past few days or week.[15] Finally, not all biologic screens test for common drugs of abuse (eg, synthetic opioids) unless special tests are requested.[15]

Although blood and urine specimens are the most common substrates for testing, other matrices, such hair, meconium, and breath samples, are undergoing evaluation and may become more widely available. The measurement of fatty acid ethyl esters in hair reflects excessive alcohol use equivalent to 4 to 29 drinks per day, but not less extreme patterns of consumption.[16] Hair samples, moreover, do not offer information about time of use.[15] Another example involving fatty acid ethyl esters is in meconium, which several studies have shown to be a biomarker of fetal ethanol exposure in the second and third trimester of pregnancy, but not the first.[14] A recent study has evaluated the use of breath samples to ascertain cannabis use for the purposes of detecting "driving under the influence" and has found a short window of detection (use within 0.5–2 hours).[17]

Finally, biologic tests examine a sample with a drug concentration at specific cutoff levels (**Table 1**). So, the implications of either a positive or negative test are not absolute. A positive test may reflect ingestion of an innocuous substance that tests like one that is problematic. A negative test may simply confirm the absence of recent use but not remote or subthreshold use.

Questionnaires

Questionnaires about the prenatal use of alcohol and other drugs may be useful in achieving consistent screening. At the time of writing, the development and evaluation of screening measures for prenatal alcohol use is well advanced, but the validity, reliability, and clinical use of standardized questionnaires in screening for illicit drug use during pregnancy is not commensurate.[10,11]

Table 1
Analytes and their cutoffs

Initial Test Analyte	Initial Test Cutoff Concentration	Confirmatory Test Analyte	Confirmatory Test Cutoff Concentration
Marijuana metabolites	50 ng/mL	THCA	15 ng/mL
Cocaine metabolites	150 ng/mL	Benzoylecgonine	100 ng/mL
Opioid metabolites Codeine/morphine[a]	2000 ng/mL	Codeine Morphine	2000 ng/mL 2000 ng/mL
6-Acetylmorphine	10 ng/mL	6-Acetylmorphine	10 ng/mL
Phencyclidine	25 ng/mL	Phencyclidine	25 ng/mL
Amphetamines[b] AMP/MAMP[c]	500 ng/mL	Amphetamine Methamphetamine[d]	250 ng/mL 250 ng/mL
MDMA	500 ng/mL	MDMA MDA MDEA	250 ng/mL 250 ng/mL 250 ng/mL

Abbreviations: MDA, methylenedioxyamphetamine; MDEA, methylenedioxyethylamphetamine; MDMA, methylenedioxymethamphetamine; THCA, delta-9-tetrahydrocannabinol-9-carboxylic acid.
  [a] Morphine is the target analyte for codeine/morphine testing.
  [b] Either a single initial test kit or multiple initial test kits may be used provided the single test kit detects each target analyte independently at the specified cutoff.
  [c] Methamphetamine is the target analyte for amphetamine/methamphetamine testing.
  [d] To be reported as positive for methamphetamine, a specimen must also contain amphetamine at a concentration equal to or greater than 100 ng/mL.
  From Analytes and their cutoffs. *Federal Register,* November 25, 2008 (73 FR 71858), Section 3.4. 2010.

Box 1
The T-ACE questions

T: Tolerance

How many drinks does it take to make you feel high? (>2 drinks = 2 points)

A: Annoyed

Have people annoyed you by criticizing your drinking? (yes = 1 point)

C: Cut down

Have you ever felt you ought to cut down on your drinking? (yes = 1 point)

E: Eye-opener

Have you ever had a drink first thing in the morning to steady your nerves or get rid of a hang-over? (yes = 1 point)

The T-ACE is considered positive with a score of 2 or more. The reported sensitivity of the T-ACE has ranged from 69% to 88% and the reported specificity has ranged from 71% to 89% among pregnant women.[10]

Adapted from Sokol RH, Martier SS, Ager JW. The T-ACE questions: practical prenatal detection of risky drinking. Am J Obstet Gynecol 1989;160:863; with permission.

Sensitivity and specificity are two important properties of every screening instrument. The sensitivity of a screening test refers to the probability that a person who should test positive, does so (ie, the sensitivity of a screen for pregnancy risk drinking is the probability that a woman who is a risk drinker tests positive). The specificity of a screening test is the probability that a person who should test negative, does so (ie, the probability that a woman who is not a risk drinker tests negative).[18]

The American College of Obstetricians and Gynecologists has created a prevention tool kit to identify risky drinking before and during pregnancy and to offer a brief intervention that could be incorporated into routine care.[19] Three steps are described: (1)

Box 2
Tweak test

Do you drink alcoholic beverages? If you do, please take the TWEAK TEST.

T: Tolerance: how many drinks can you hold?

W: Have close friends or relatives worried or complained about your drinking in the past year?

E: Eye-opener: Do you sometimes take a drink in the morning when you first get up?

A: Amnesia (Blackouts) has a friend or family member ever told you about things you said or did while you were drinking that you could not remember?

K: Do you sometimes feel the need to cut down on your drinking?

To score the test, a seven point scale is used. The tolerance question is scored two points if a woman reports that she can hold more than 5 drinks without passing out. A positive response to the worry question yields two points. A yes to any of the remaining questions scores one point for each positive response. The TWEAK is positive with a score of 3 or more and suggests that the woman is likely to be a heavy/problem drinker. The reported sensitivity of the TWEAK has ranged from 71% to 91% and the reported specificity has ranged from 73% to 83% among pregnant women.[10]

From Russell M, Martier SS, Sokol RJ, et al. Screening for pregnancy risk drinking: TWEAKING the tests. Alcohol Clin Exp Res 1991;15:638; with permission.

Box 3
Alcohol Use Disorders Identification Test–Consumption

1. How often did you have a drink containing alcohol in the past year?

   Never (0 points, If you answered never, score questions 2 and 3 as zero)

   Monthly or less (1 point)

   2 to 4 times a month (2 points)

   2 or 3 times per week (3 points)

   4 or more times a week (4 points)

2. How many drinks did you have on a typical day when you were drinking in the past year?

   1 or 2 (0 points)

   3 or 4 (1 point)

   5 or 6 (2 points)

   7 to 9 (3 points)

   10 or more (4 points)

3. How often did you have 6 or more drinks on one occasion in the past year?

   Never (0 points)

   Less than monthly (1 point)

   Monthly (2 points)

   Weekly (3 points)

   Daily or almost daily (4 points)

The Alcohol Use Disorders Identification Test–Consumption (AUDIT-C) is scored on a scale of 0 to 12 (a score of 0 reflects no alcohol use). A score of 3 or more in women is considered positive and suggests the need for further evaluation. Generally, the higher the AUDIT-C score, the more likely it is that the patient's drinking is affecting his or her health and safety. Reported sensitivity has been about 95% and reported specificity has been about 85% among pregnant women.[10]

Adapted from Bush K, Kivlahan DR, McDonnell MB, et al. The AUDIT alcohol consumption questions (UAIDT-C): an effective brief screening test for problem drinking. Ambulatory Care Quality Improvement Project (ACQUIP). Alcohol Use Disorders Identification Test. Arch Intern Med 1998;158:1790; with permission.

---

ask about alcohol use, (2) brief intervention, and (3) follow-up. If a patient answers "yes" to the question, "have you ever had a drink containing alcohol," then administering a validated screening tool is recommended. The T-ACE is one such example (**Box 1**). Other screening questionnaires have also been tested among pregnant women; the TWEAK and Alcohol Use Disorders Identification Test–Consumption are among the most promising (**Boxes 2 and 3**).[10]

Screening tools for prenatal drug use are available but have not been as extensively studied. At the time of writing, several tools seem to be promising but have limitations, such as lack of validation in larger or different samples. The Substance Use Risk Profile–Pregnancy Scale asks three yes/no questions that yield an estimate of risk of prenatal drug use.[20] The estimated sensitivity (91%) and specificity (67%) have been reported, based on a validation study including 1074 women. The Substance Use Risk Profile–Pregnancy Scale questions are listed in **Box 4**.

Box 4
Substance use risk profile–pregnancy scale

1. Have you ever smoked marijuana?

2. In the month before you knew you were pregnant, how many beers, how much wine, or how much liquor did you drink?

3. Have you ever felt that you needed to cut down on your drug or alcohol use?

Scoring information:

Classify the number of alcoholic drinks before pregnancy as none compared with any. Count the number of affirmative items.

0 = low risk

1 = moderate risk

2–3 = high risk

In low-risk populations, one or more affirmative items indicate a positive screen, whereas in high-risk populations, two or more affirmative items indicate a positive screen.

Adapted from Yonkers KA, Gotman N, Kershaw T, et al. Screening for prenatal substance use: development of the substance use risk profile–pregnancy scale. Obstet Gynecol 2010;116: 831; with permission.

The 4Ps family of screening tools is popular and began in 1990.[21] Since then, the measure has evolved along two paths. The first path is to the 4Ps Plus, which is copyrighted and not perceived to be freely available for use without charge. The second path has been to the 5Ps Prenatal Substance Abuse Screen for Alcohol and Drugs, as adapted by the Massachusetts Institute for Health and Recovery.[22] Although reported to be in wide use in Massachusetts, California, Maine, Virginia, and South Carolina, the 5Ps has not been subject to rigorous, systematic study (no comparison with a criterion standard, no calculation of measures of merit). The 5Ps consist of five yes/no questions, listed in **Box 5**.

There is some previous research comparing questionnaires against physiologic markers of drug use during pregnancy. One study compared the DAST-10 with urine

---

Box 5
The 5Ps

1. Did any of your Parents have a problem with alcohol or drug use?

2. Do you any of your friends (Peers) have a problem with alcohol or other drug use?

3. Does your Partner have a problem with alcohol or drug use?

4. Before you were pregnant did you have a problem with alcohol or use (Past)?

5. In the month before you knew you were pregnant, did you drink any beer, wine, or liquor, or use other drugs including marijuana and prescription drugs taken other than directed (Pregnancy)?

A single "yes" suggests further assessment. This screener has no reported measures of merit (eg, sensitivity, specificity).

Adapted from Watson E. Institute on Health and Recovery, Integrated Screening Tool. Cambridge (MA). Available at: http://www.mhqp.org/guidelines/perinatalPDF/IHRIntegratedScreeningTool. pdf. Accessed February 5, 2014; with permission.

and hair samples in a sample of 300 low-income, postpartum women. The DAST-10 is a 10-item measure of consequences related to drug use. Twenty-four percent of the sample scored positive on the DAST but had negative toxicology results, whereas 19% of the sample had positive toxicology results but denied drug use on the DAST. Measures of merit of the DAST-10 (with the cutoff score of 1) for any drug use were sensitivity of 0.47, specificity of 0.82, positive predictive value of 0.43, and negative predictive value of 0.84.[23]

SUMMARY AND RECOMMENDATIONS

The use of alcohol and other substances is not infrequent during pregnancy and has been associated with adverse effects on pregnancy outcome. Although pregnant women have been described to be highly motivated to change their behaviors in their pursuit of healthful practices, they may not routinely discuss their use of alcohol and other drugs.[24] As such, prenatal health care providers may wish to screen all pregnant patients for their use of alcohol and other drugs using an approach that works best in their setting.

A positive screen is not a diagnosis. Rather, it is an opportunity for the clinician and patient to discuss health practices and behaviors, such as the use of alcohol and other drugs in the antepartum. The discussion may lead the clinician to refer the patient for further assessment or offer a brief intervention or other types of support during the time leading up to delivery.

This article highlights the limitations of currently available tools to identify prenatal alcohol and drug use. Future research should prioritize the validation of efficient and effective screening methods to optimize pregnancy outcomes.

REFERENCES

1. Substance Abuse and Mental Health Services Administration. Results from the 2012 National Survey on Drug Use and Health: summary of national findings. NSDUH Series H-46, HHS Publication No. (SMA) 13–4795. Rockville (MD): Substance Abuse and Mental Health Services Administration; 2013.
2. Patrick SW, Schumacher RE, Benneyworth BD, et al. Neonatal abstinence syndrome and associated health care expenditures. JAMA 2012;307:1934–40.
3. Hayes MJ, Brown MS. Epidemic of prescription opiate abuse and neonatal abstinence. JAMA 2012;307:1974–5.
4. Keyes KM, Grant BF, Hasin DS. Evidence for a closing gender gap in alcohol use, abuse, and dependence in the United States population. Drug Alcohol Depend 2008;93:21–9.
5. Ethen MK, Ramadhani TA, Scheherle AE, et al. National birth defects prevention study. Matern Child Health J 2007;13:274–85.
6. Zizzo N, DiPietro N, Green C, et al. Comments and reflections on ethics in screening for biomarkers of prenatal alcohol exposure. Alcohol Clin Exp Res 2013;37(9):1451–5. http://dx.doi.org/10.1111/acer.12115.
7. American College of Obstetricians and Gynecologists. At-risk drinking and illicit drug use: ethical issues in obstetric and gynecologic practice. ACOG Committee Opinion No. 422. Obstet Gynecol 2008;112:1449–60.
8. Svikis DS, Reid-Quinones K. Screening and prevention of alcohol and drug use disorders in women. Obstet Gynecol Clin North Am 2003;30:447–68.
9. American College of Obstetricians and Gynecologists. Committee on Health Care for Underserved Women. Substance abuse reporting and pregnancy: the role of

the obstetrician-gynecologist. Committee Opinion No. 473. Obstet Gynecol 2011; 117:200–1.

10. Burns E, Gray R, Smith LA. Brief screening questionnaires to identify problem drinking during pregnancy: a systematic review. Addiction 2010;105:611–4.

11. US Preventive Services Task Force. Screening for illicit drug use: US Preventive services task force recommendation statement. 2008. Available at: http://www.uspreventiveservicestaskforce.org/uspstf08/druguse/drugrs.htm. Accessed March 13, 2014.

12. US Preventive Services Task Force. Counseling and interventions to prevent tobacco use and tobacco-caused disease in adults and pregnant women: US Preventive Services Task Force Reaffirmation Recommendation Statement. Ann Intern Med 2009;150:551–5.

13. US Preventive Services Task Force. USPSTF A and B recommendations. Available at: http://www.uspreventiveservicestaskforce.org/uspstf/uspsabrecs.htm. Accessed March 13, 2014.

14. Joya X, Friguls B, Ortigosa S, et al. Determination of maternal-fetal biomarkers of prenatal exposure to ethanol: a review. J Pharm Biomed Anal 2012;69:209–22.

15. National Institute on Drug Abuse. Resource guide: screening for drug use in general medical settings. Available at: http://www.drugabuse.gov/publications/resource-guide/biological-specimen-testing. Accessed January 13, 2014.

16. Kulaga V, Shor S, Loren G. Correlation between drugs of abuse and alcohol by hair analysis: parents at risk for having children with fetal alcohol spectrum disorder. Alcohol 2010;44:615–21.

17. Himes SK, Scheidweiler KB, Beck O, et al. Cannabinoids in exhaled breath following controlled administration of smoked cannabis. Clin Chem 2013; 59(12):1780–9. http://dx.doi.org/10.1373/clinchem.2013.207407.

18. Rosner B. Fundamentals of biostatistics. Belmont (CA): Duxbury Press; 1990. p. 55.

19. American College of Obstetricians and Gynecologists. Drinking and reproductive health. A fetal alcohol spectrum disorders prevention tool kit. Available at: http://www.acog.org/. Accessed January 12, 2014.

20. Yonkers KA, Gotman N, Kershaw T, et al. Screening for prenatal substance use: development of the substance use risk profile–pregnancy scale. Obstet Gynecol 2010;116:827–33.

21. Ewing H. A practical guide to intervention in health and social services, with pregnant and post-partum addicts and alcoholics. The Born Free Project.

22. Watson E. Institute on Health and Recovery. Cambridge (MA).

23. Grekin ER, Svikis DS, Lam P, et al. Drug use during pregnancy: validating the drug abuse screening test against physiological measures. Psychol Addict Behav 2011;24:719–29.

24. Hankin J, McCaul ME, Heussner J. Pregnant, alcohol-abusing women. Alcohol Clin Exp Res 2000;24:1276–86.

Prenatal and Postpartum Care of Women with Substance Use Disorders

Sarah Gopman, BA, MD

KEYWORDS

- Prenatal care • Substance abuse disorder • Postpartum care • Opioid dependence
- Opioid replacement therapy • Pregnancy • Opioid addiction

KEY POINTS

- Prenatal care providers should screen all patients for substance abuse disorders in pregnancy using a validated screening tool.
- Women identified as having a substance abuse disorder in pregnancy should be offered coordinated multidisciplinary care.
- Opioid replacement therapy improves pregnancy outcomes for women with opioid dependence and is not a contraindication to breastfeeding.
- Women with substance abuse disorders should be evaluated and treated for concurrent psychiatric disorders.
- A respectful, nonjudgmental, and flexible approach by clinicians encourages ongoing patient participation in prenatal care.

INTRODUCTION
Epidemiology of Substance Abuse in Pregnancy

The use of substances of abuse in pregnancy creates significant barriers to receiving high-quality prenatal, intrapartum, and postpartum care (**Box 1**). Yet clinicians who recognize and directly face this challenge have an opportunity to make a substantial impact on perinatal outcomes and the long-term health of women and their children. The incidence of substance abuse among pregnant women reflects that of the general population and nonpregnant women by age group. Data from the 2012 National Survey on Drug Use and Health shows that the rate of current illicit drug use among girls and women aged 12 or older was 6.9%. This survey also determined that among girls and women ages 15 to 44, encompassing the reproductive years, 10.7% of nonpregnant women and 5.9% of pregnant women were current illicit drug users, based on

The author has nothing to disclose.
Family and Community Medicine, University of New Mexico, MSC09-5040, 2400 Tucker Avenue, Northeast, Albuquerque, NM 87131, USA
E-mail address: sgopman@salud.unm.edu

> **Box 1**
> **Barriers to care for pregnant women with substance use disorders**
>
> - Inadequate screening for substance abuse by prenatal care providers
> - Fear of seeking care due to societal stigma and legal ramifications
> - High baseline anxiety and poor coping skills
> - Difficulty establishing trusting relationships with providers
> - Underlying psychiatric disorders
> - Lack of transportation and child care
> - Intimate partner violence and/or controlling behavior of partner
> - Incarceration

averaging of data from 2011 and 2012. Analysis of pregnancy-related data by age group shows that, among pregnant teens ages 15 to 17, the rate of current illicit drug use was 18.3% and was 9.0% for pregnant women ages 18 to 25 and 3.4% among those aged 26 to 44.[1]

Opioids account for a substantial proportion of substances abused, with disturbing trends toward increased use in recent years, including illicit opioids, such as heroin, and prescription opioids, such as oxycodone. A study analyzing *International Classification of Diseases, Ninth Revision, Clinical Modification* codes showed an increase in antepartum maternal opioid use from 1.19 to 5.63 per 1000 hospital births between the years 2000 and 2009.[2] During the same period, the incidence of neonatal abstinence syndrome (NAS) increased from 1.20 to 3.39 infants per 1000 hospital births.[2] This study also assessed costs related to the treatment of NAS, which were estimated at a mean of $53,400 per infant hospitalization in 2009.[2]

Effects of Substance Abuse on Pregnancy

Pregnancies complicated by substance abuse are at risk of miscarriage, preterm delivery, intrauterine growth restriction, placental abruption, fetal intraventricular hemorrhage, intrauterine fetal demise, NAS, and other infant developmental effects.[3] An accurate accounting of total costs related to substance abuse in pregnancy would need to include those related to antepartum hospitalizations for drug intoxication, withdrawal, and associated complications; correctional services expenditures related to incarceration and associated legal costs; care of infants born prematurely or with other medical complications related to substance exposure; funding of child protective services investigations and interventions; and the essentially impossible-to-quantify cost of human suffering of women and their children, families, and communities.

CHALLENGES FOR CLINICIANS
Appropriate Screening Implementation

Given the incidence of substance abuse in pregnancy, all clinicians who provide prenatal care encounter affected women, regardless of practice setting and demographic characteristics. Care is complicated by the difficulty of identifying women with substance abuse issues in pregnancy. Clinicians may fail to appropriately screen patients due to concerns about time utilization, the belief that their practice setting does not include women with substance abuse issues, or lack of resources available for those who screen positive.[4] Although universal urine drug screening has been advocated by some clinicians and policy makers, this practice fails to identify women with sporadic but clinically significant use[5] and may discourage women from seeking prenatal care. Urine drug testing based on clinician suspicion risks racial and socioeconomic profiling. Several validated survey-type screening tools are available, including the 4 Ps,[4] T-ACE,[6] TWEAK,[7] and others,[4] and these provide an efficient and effective means of screening all pregnancies for substance abuse (**Box 2**). These tools can

---

Box 2
Screening tools for substance use disorders in pregnancy

TWEAK[a]

T: Tolerance—How many drinks can you hold?

W: Have close friends or relatives *Worried* or complained about your drinking in the past year?

E: Eye-opener—Do you sometimes take a drink in the morning when you first get up?

A: Amnesia—Has a friend or family member ever told you about things you said or did while you were drinking that you could not remember?

K(C): Do you sometimes feel the need to *Cut down* on your drinking:

A 7-point scale is used to score the test. The Tolerance question scores 2 points if a woman reports she can hold more than 5 drinks without falling asleep or passing out. A positive response to the Worried question scores 2 points, and a positive response to the last 3 questions scores 1 point each. A total score of 2 or more points indicates the woman is likely to be a risk drinker.

T-ACE[b]

T: Tolerance—How many drinks does it take to make you feel high?

A positive answer, scored a 2, is more than 2 drinks. This suggests tolerance of alcohol and very likely a history of at least moderate alcohol intake.

A: Annoyed—Have people annoyed you by criticizing your drinking?

C: Cut down—Have you felt you ought to cut down on your drinking?

E: Eve opener—Have you ever had a drink first thing in the morning to steady your nerves or get rid of a hangover?

The first question is scored 0 or 2 points. The last 3 questions are scored 1 point if answered affirmatively. A total score of 2 or more is considered positive for risk drinking.

4 Ps[c]

Have you ever used drugs or alcohol during this *Pregnancy*?

Have you had a problem with drugs or alcohol in the *Past*?

Does your *Partner* have a problem with drugs or alcohol?

Do you consider one of your *Parents* to be an addict or alcoholic?

This screening device is often used as a way to begin a discussion about drug or alcohol use. Any woman who answers yes to one or more questions should be referred for further assessment.

[a] *From* Russell M. New assessment tools for drinking in pregnancy: T-ACE, TWEAK, and others. Alcohol Health Res World 1994;18:59.
[b] *Adapted from* Sokol RJ, Martier SS, Ager JW. The T-ACE questions: practical prenatal detection of risk-drinking. Am J Obstet Gynecol 1989;160(4):865.
[c] *From* Ewing H. A practical guide to intervention in health and social services, with pregnant and postpartum addicts and alcoholics. Martinez, CA: The Born Free Project, Contra Costa County Department of Health Service; 1990.

be effectively administered in a few minutes during a prenatal intake appointment. Those who screen positive require a more detailed assessment of their substance abuse disorder.

Societal Stigma and Patient Fears

Pregnant women with substance abuse disorders face stigmatization and judgment from society and the medical profession, despite that many women arrive at substance abuse after victimization via childhood sexual abuse or neglect, adult sexual assault, intimate partner violence, and prostitution as well as mental health disorders.[8] Clinicians who provide specialized care to this patient population may find the need to educate colleagues and other staff members regarding these risk factors and the need for sensitivity and compassion.[4]

Women with substance abuse disorders are often afraid to seek prenatal care due to concerns about legal ramifications, including involvement of child protective services.[9] Because of these fears, they may present to care late in the pregnancy or fail to seek care until the onset of pregnancy complication symptoms or labor. They may have difficulty establishing trusting relationships with their prenatal care providers, which can impede their ability to discuss important aspects of their health. In addition, substance abuse charges account for a large proportion of women who are incarcerated,[10] and those who are pregnant and jailed face significant challenges in accessing appropriate prenatal care[11] and substance abuse treatment, including difficulties obtaining opioid replacement therapy.[12] When women are released from incarceration, provisions may not be made for ongoing prenatal care, including failure to convey information from the correctional facility to the women about upcoming scheduled prenatal care and related appointments.

High Resource Utilization

Caring for women with substance abuse disorders in pregnancy is resource intensive. Women may require more frequent appointments and may miss more appointments due to transportation difficulties and lack of child care compared to women without substance abuse disorders.[9,13] High baseline anxiety levels, poor coping skills, and underlying psychiatric disorders[14] can require more clinician time during prenatal care appointments to adequately support women and promote trust and confidence in care providers. Multidisciplinary care, including using substance abuse counselors, social workers, case managers, psychiatrists, and opioid replacement therapy providers, is required for optimization of care.[15]

PRENATAL MANAGEMENT
Pregnancy Options Counseling

Women with active substance abuse disorders are at risk for unplanned pregnancy.[16] On diagnosis of pregnancy, a woman's feelings about being pregnant and about parenting should be elicited and pregnancy options counseling should be provided if desired. A discussion of pregnancy options includes information about parenting, adoption, and pregnancy termination via medication or surgical abortion.

Substance Abuse History, Patient Education, and Harm Reduction

Once substance use is identified using a recommended screening tool or due to patient disclosure, a thorough substance abuse history should be taken. This includes identifying which substances are used, plus the route (inhalation, ingestion, or injection), frequency, and length of use. Symptoms that occur on discontinuation of the substance should be reviewed to determine whether dependence exists, which results in a withdrawal syndrome. The substance use history of close family members and partner(s) should also be elicited. Women should be educated about the risks of individual substances to their health and the health of the pregnancy, including risks related to alcohol and tobacco use. Many patients decrease their use of substances of abuse to some degree simply after a discussion of risks with their health care provider.[4]

Substance abuse disorder is a relapsing-remitting condition. During treatment, periods of abstinence are interrupted by relapse to use of the substance(s) of abuse, followed by a return to abstinence. The goal is for periods of abstinence to become longer, with relapses becoming shorter in duration and further apart. A harm reduction approach recognizes the likelihood of relapse and encourages ongoing care even when relapse occurs.[17] This requires creating an environment in which women feel safe and do not fear condemnation and criticism when they divulge the occurrence of a relapse.[18]

Opioid Replacement Therapy

General benefits
High-quality evidence from the medical literature demonstrates that individuals with opioid dependence are most likely to remain free of relapse to substances of abuse when they receive treatment with opioid replacement therapy.[19] Agents available for use in the United States include methadone and buprenorphine. Both are long-acting opioids that allow a steady serum opioid level without periods of intoxication and withdrawal, thereby decreasing associated health risks. They treat opioid withdrawal and decrease or eliminate drug cravings.[20] In doing so, they may help patients avoid dangerous activities associated with drug use, including sharing needles, exchanging sex for drugs, engaging in crimes to obtain money to purchase drugs, and falling victim to violence in the process of obtaining drugs. They also prevent overdose deaths caused by opioids of abuse.[21] In freeing patients from time spent in activities associated with obtaining and using substances of abuse, they allow time to re-establish focus on healthy goals, such as parenting, education, and employment.[18]

Benefits in pregnancy
The specific benefits of opioid replacement therapy in pregnancy include avoiding the cycles of intoxication and withdrawal that are common in those with dependence on short-acting opioids, such as heroin or oxycodone, thereby avoiding the effects of these cycles on the fetus, including preterm delivery, intrauterine growth restriction, and intrauterine fetal demise.[22] Opioid replacement therapy is also associated with longer gestation[23] and higher infant birth weight.[24]

Methadone and buprenorphine
Options for opioid replacement therapy in pregnancy include both methadone and buprenorphine. Methadone is a pure opioid agonist available through federally approved facilities that dispense daily oral liquid doses to patients initially, with the option to provide take-home doses as the period of adherence to the treatment plan lengthens. It is increased slowly over the course of weeks to achieve a therapeutic level and can cause respiratory depression and death if the dose is increased too quickly. Buprenorphine is a mixed opioid agonist-antagonist available by prescription from physicians who have participated in special training and have received a license from the Drug Enforcement Agency to prescribe it. It is administered sublingually when used for opioid replacement therapy. Because of its strong affinity for the opioid receptor but only partial activation of the receptor, patients must be in at least moderate

opioid withdrawal at the time it is initiated to avoid precipitated opioid withdrawal (i.e. buprenorphine displaces other opioids from the opioid receptor but does not activate the receptor as completely as pure opioid agonists, thus causing opioid withdrawal in opioid dependent individuals whose receptors are still "filled" with another opioid). Once the patient enters moderate opioid withdrawal, an initial dose of buprenorphine is given, symptoms are monitored, and additional doses are given every few hours in order to control withdrawal symptoms and opioid cravings. A therapeutic dose is generally reached in 24 hours or less. In adults, buprenorphine shows a ceiling effect with respect to respiratory depression that reduces the risk of overdose death.[25]

Use of opioid replacement therapy should continue throughout pregnancy and for at least several months postpartum to reduce risk of relapse.[26] Many patients are best treated with long-term maintenance of opioid replacement therapy over the course of several years due to a history of relapse during prior attempts at weaning or discontinuing medication.[27] Clinicians who provide prenatal care and are not licensed and trained to prescribe buprenorphine in pregnancy can establish collaborative relationships with those who manage opioid replacement therapy to facilitate care.

For pregnant women with significant opioid dependence, weaning opioids or quitting use abruptly to achieve abstinence is not recommended, because opioid withdrawal may increase the risk of miscarriage, preterm labor, fetal distress, and intrauterine fetal demise and most commonly results in relapse.[28] Some women may decline opioid replacement therapy or may not have access to it due to their geographic location remote from trained providers of this service. A recent retrospective cohort study of 95 women who chose detoxification from opioids and underwent an inpatient methadone wean showed a 56% success rate when defined as no maternal illicit opioid use at the time of delivery as determined by maternal report, maternal urine drug toxicology, or newborn meconium toxicology.[29] Information was not provided in this study regarding longer-term outcomes of women and their infants. Medically supervised opioid detoxification can be considered in select and highly motivated pregnant patients, but is associated with a high rate of relapse to opioids of abuse.

All opioids, including opioid replacement therapies, cause slower gastrointestinal motility, resulting in significant constipation for many patients.[30] Women may discontinue use of prenatal vitamins due to the additional constipating effect of the iron contained in them, and appetite can be poor in those with chronic constipation. Patients may be reluctant to discuss this problem with their prenatal care provider, although it is usually readily treated with twice-daily use of stool softeners, such as docusate, plus osmotic agents, such as polyethylene glycol, when needed. Clinicians should inquire about constipation symptoms when caring for women with opioid dependence.[31]

Neonatal abstinence syndrome

Women should be informed that infants exposed to opioids in utero, whether substances of abuse or opioid replacement therapy, require observation and treatment, if indicated, for NAS. Newborns are observed for 3 to 7 days for development of NAS, and those who require pharmacologic treatment are generally administered oral morphine or methadone (although other agents are sometimes used).[32] Once a dose is achieved that effectively ameliorates signs and symptoms of opioid withdrawal, the dose is weaned over several days and then discontinued, with a period of observation after the last dose to assure clinical stability. Infants of women who are treated with buprenorphine may have less risk of requiring pharmacologic treatment of NAS, and treatment periods may be shorter in duration.[33]

Counseling and Support

A key component of substance abuse treatment includes counseling. Where possible, this is best provided by individuals with specialized training in treatment of substance abuse. Counselors and substance abuse treatment programs may use a variety of techniques, including motivational interviewing, identification of triggers for relapse, stress reduction education, meditation, cognitive behavioral therapy, positive reinforcement of abstinence, contingency management, and support groups.[34] Alternative therapies, such as acupuncture, may also be offered. Patients may be encouraged to develop a new social network to avoid contact with acquaintances, friends, and family members who continue in the drug lifestyle.

Evaluation and Treatment of Associated Health Conditions

Women with substance abuse disorders often suffer from a lack of general health care prior to the pregnancy.[35] They may have higher risks for certain health conditions and diseases, including tobacco use, sexually transmitted infections (STIs), hepatitis C, and HIV.[26] Dental health may be neglected during periods of active drug use.[36] Underlying mental health disorders, such as depression, anxiety, posttraumatic stress disorder (PTSD), bipolar disorder, schizophrenia, and personality disorders, may go undiagnosed or untreated.

Tobacco addiction

Use of tobacco in pregnancy is associated with increased risk of ectopic gestation, abnormal placentation, intrauterine growth restriction, preterm delivery, and sudden infant death syndrome.[37] Although clinicians understandably focus significant attention on discontinuation of illicit substances and alcohol in pregnancy, smoking cessation is an important goal. Nicotine replacement products may be considered, although concerns exist about their use in pregnancy.[38] Helping women identify triggers for smoking, setting a quit date, encouraging partners to stop smoking, and offering positive reinforcement for efforts to decrease use are all appropriate measures.[39,40]

Sexually transmitted infections and hepatitis C

In addition to standard prenatal laboratory studies, including STI testing, screening for the hepatitis C antibody should be performed. Those who test positive for the hepatitis C antibody should have polymerase chain reaction testing to evaluate viral load and liver function tests to assess for evidence of liver inflammation/injury. Elevated transaminases can be followed serially, and any evidence for worsening while on buprenorphine for opioid replacement therapy should be noted and therapy altered if indicated.[27] Acetaminophen, although generally considered safe in pregnancy, should be used sparingly by those with underlying liver disease; although definitive studies are lacking, a maximum of 2000 mg per day is thought safe.[41] Consideration should be given for repeating STI and hepatitis C screening in the third trimester, depending on relapse to substances of abuse and/or other risk factors.[22]

Dental disease

An oral examination may identify obvious caries or periodontal disease, and dental referral can facilitate routine cleanings to maintain dental health during pregnancy as well as address active disease. A letter from a referring clinician outlining acceptable dental care in pregnancy may reassure dental professionals of the appropriateness of proceeding with treatment when indicated.[42]

Psychiatric disorders

Brief self-administered mental health surveys, such as the Patient Health Questionnaire (PHQ-9) for depression and the Mood Disorder Questionnaire (MDQ) for bipolar disorder, are designed for screening purposes and can be used in the prenatal care setting.[43] Women with a self-reported history or who screen positive for mental health disorders require further assessment. Active use of substances of abuse may interfere with assessment of psychiatric disorders; therefore, a period of stability on opioid replacement therapy or abstinence from stimulants and/or other psychoactive drugs may be needed prior to verification of underlying psychiatric diagnoses.[26] Anxiety and PTSD are also prevalent among women with substance abuse disorders. When psychiatric disorders are found, discussion of treatment options should be undertaken, and the use of pharmacologic treatments should not be withheld simply because of pregnancy. After adequate patient counseling about risks and benefits of pharmacologic treatment, some medications may be appropriate for the prenatal care provider to prescribe without further consultation with a psychiatric professional, including serotonin reuptake inhibitors for depression and sedating antihistamines, such as hydroxyzine for anxiety.[44] Care should be taken to discuss any new medications with providers managing opioid replacement therapy to ensure safety in combination. Decisions regarding treatment with mood stabilizers and antipsychotics are less likely to be undertaken by prenatal care providers without psychiatric consultation.

Environmental stressors

Assessment of social and environmental stressors is indicated for all pregnancies; however, women with substance abuse disorders may be at higher risk for these problems. Screening for issues such as intimate partner violence, homelessness, and food insecurity, should be performed routinely on initial presentation, periodically over the course of prenatal care, and when changes in social circumstances occur. These assessments are best performed privately and confidentially[26] and are facilitated by routinely asking family members and partners to leave the examination room for a period of time at each visit, thus normalizing the practice. Women who do not have a safe and supportive living environment that is free of substance abuse and other dangers or who require more intensive management may be helped by residential treatment.[45] Ideally, these programs provide housing, case management, substance abuse counseling, group therapy, and parenting education and support.

Anticipating Absences from Care

Late presentation to prenatal care may stem from fear of seeking care, a chaotic lifestyle associated with active drug use, transportation and child care issues, and controlling or abusive partners.[9] Flexibility in appointment scheduling, including the ability to see women for care on short notice and the willingness to see them despite late arrivals for appointments, can facilitate entry into substance abuse treatment and more complete prenatal care.[46] Anticipating the possibility of fewer total prenatal care appointments or future missed appointments allows clinicians to prioritize important assessments. For example, a brief ultrasound in the office for confirmation of pregnancy dating at the initial visit can provide information crucial for later medical decision making in the event that a patient is subsequently absent from care for a prolonged period of time.

Assessing Fetal Well-Being

Although opioid replacement therapy is associated with improved pregnancy outcomes in women with opioid dependence, some evidence suggests lower birth weights for infants exposed to methadone in utero. Similar trends have not been noted for buprenorphine use in pregnancy.[47] Careful assessment of fetal growth via serial fundal height measurements is indicated. Although evidence is lacking, consideration can be given for ultrasound assessment of fetal growth, for example, at 28 and 34 weeks' gestational age. Ongoing use of substances of abuse, in particular stimulants, is associated with an increased risk of intrauterine growth restriction and perinatal death.[48–51] One approach is to institute weekly fetal heart rate monitoring at 32 weeks' gestational age for women with ongoing use of stimulants[52] and to consider induction of labor at 38 weeks' gestational age, balancing risks of induction with risks of continued stimulant exposure.

Supporting Preparation for Parenting

By accessing prenatal care and disclosing substance abuse, women are taking the first of many potential steps toward improving their health and investing in the health of their children and families. The courage required to do so is particularly striking in cases of women who have grown up in families afflicted by generations of substance abuse.[53] They may be motivated by their own experiences of neglect or abuse in their families of origin or by experiences as children in the foster care system but may have few examples of healthy parenting to emulate as they raise their own children. Assistance in preparing for parenthood is key for women and their partners in these circumstances, and referrals to educational programs should be provided.[54] Preparation for parenting also includes education regarding NAS and its diagnosis and treatment, including expected length of hospital stay for the infant.

BRIEF OVERVIEW OF INTRAPARTUM MANAGEMENT

Labor management for women with substance abuse does not differ greatly from routine care. Continuous fetal heart rate monitoring can be considered due to uncertain effects of previous substance exposures on the ability of the fetus to tolerate labor. Baseline fetal heart rate may be lower in women who are treated with methadone and decreased reactivity may be noted for 2 to 3 hours after a methadone dose; this effect is less prominent in women treated with buprenorphine.[55]

The use of a fetal scalp electrode for fetal heart rate monitoring should be avoided if possible in women with hepatitis C, although a recent systematic review was inconclusive on the relationship to vertical transmission of hepatitis C.[56] The use of internal fetal monitoring should also be avoided in patients with HIV.[57]

Women may present for the first time in labor without previous prenatal care, and opioid-dependent women may exhibit opioid withdrawal during this time. Methadone or buprenorphine can be initiated during labor, although buprenorphine must be dosed at a therapeutic level before other opioids are used for pain control in this situation due to risk of precipitated withdrawal if buprenorphine is initiated while opioid withdrawal symptoms are mitigated by other opioid pain medications.

Opioid replacement therapy should be continued during labor, including giving any doses that are due during that time.[58] Although intravenous opioids at typical doses may be less-effective labor analgesia for women on opioid replacement therapy, pure opioid agonists are not contraindicated for women on stable doses of methadone or buprenorphine as long as there is no evidence of oversedation in association with their use. Mixed agonist-antagonists, such as nalbuphine, butorphanol, and pentazocine, can precipitate withdrawal in opioid-dependent individuals and should be avoided. Obtaining venous access in patients with a history of intravenous substance abuse can be challenging and may require additional time and/or advanced techniques. Epidural anesthesia is a good choice if pharmacologic pain management is desired. Patients undergoing scheduled cesarean section should continue opioid replacement therapy, including on the day of delivery. The choice of whether to use long-acting opioids in spinal or epidural anesthetics placed for cesarean section varies among anesthesiologists.[59]

POSTPARTUM MANAGEMENT
Pain Management

Postpartum pain management for patients who deliver vaginally can usually be achieved without the use of opioid pain medications. Non-steroidal anti-inflammatory drugs (NSAIDs) and acetaminophen are typically sufficient. In the immediate postoperative period after cesarean section, higher doses of intravenous or oral opioids may be needed for pain control in women with opioid tolerance.[59] In women using buprenorphine, this need may be due to the strong affinity but only partial activation of the opioid receptor, thereby limiting access to the receptor for other opioid pain medications.[59] Opioid-dependent women may also have poorer pain tolerance due to chronic alterations in pain pathways.[60] Consideration can be given for dividing the usual buprenorphine dose in 4-times-a-day administration to contribute to postoperative pain management.

A reasonable approach is to allow for higher and/or more frequent doses of oral opioids in the early postoperative period; provide prescriptions at the time of hospital discharge balancing this need and the expectation of decreased use by the end of the first postoperative week; and schedule an early postpartum clinic visit for 7 to 10 days after discharge from the hospital. Appropriate use of NSAIDs and acetaminophen should be emphasized during the postoperative period. Explicit discussion with patients of postoperative pain management plans helps clarify expectations and ameliorate fears of inadequate pain control.[60]

Preventing Relapse

The postpartum period is a high-risk time for relapse to substances of abuse, perhaps in part because use is no longer inhibited by maternal concerns about exposure of the fetus but also likely related to increased stress levels caused by sleep deprivation, hormonal changes, and the demands of parenting. Postpartum depression, which occurs more frequently among women with substance abuse disorders,[61] may be another risk factor for relapse.[62] Close follow-up, including an early postpartum clinic visit at 1 to 2 weeks after delivery, is recommended. At this visit, a formal assessment for postpartum depression, such as the Edinburgh Postnatal Depression Scale, can be administered, and clinicians should ask directly about drug cravings and relapse to substances of abuse.

Breastfeeding Guidance

Both methadone and buprenorphine are acceptable for use in breastfeeding mothers.[63] The amount of both drugs present in breast milk is considered unlikely to produce adverse effects in the newborn[64,65] but also unlikely to prevent or treat NAS. The act of breastfeeding and skin-to-skin contact with mother, however, may diminish some symptoms of NAS.[66,67] Breastfeeding may be a motivating factor for mothers in maintaining abstinence from substances of abuse and is shown to improve maternal-infant bonding. Many women, as well as their partners and families, erroneously assume that they cannot breastfeed while on opioid replacement therapy, and proper education during the prenatal period is indicated to dispel this myth and convey the benefits of breastfeeding. Similar beliefs exist among patients and their family members regarding hepatitis C, although this is not a contraindication to breast-feeding[56] unless nipples are cracked and bleeding. In this case, milk should be expressed and discarded until the cracked nipples have healed, and then breastfeed-ing should resume. Women who have not achieved abstinence from substances of abuse, in particular those with ongoing use of stimulants and/or alcohol, should be discouraged from breastfeeding due to risk of infant exposure via breast milk.[63] HIV is a contraindication to breastfeeding in the United States due to risk of HIV transmis-sion to the newborn and availability of other appropriate nutritional sources for infants.[68]

Newborn Developmental Assessment and Support

Families who are in recovery from substance abuse require additional support to assure stability and ongoing ability to parent. Provision of comprehensive pediatric care and case management with emphasis on developmental assessment and support are key. Programs that integrate prenatal care, substance abuse treatment, case management, child development support, and primary care for families after delivery may facilitate greater ongoing participation and trust.[69,70] When integrated care is not available, developing collaborative relationships with pediatric care providers can facilitate better transition and communication surrounding potential developmental issues in the substance-exposed newborn. Parenting classes and support groups provide opportunities for families to share knowledge and experience.[71]

Postpartum Contraception

Postpartum contraceptive plans should be addressed during the prenatal care period.[72] Unless permanent sterilization is desired, long-acting reversible contraception should be encouraged because of the low likelihood of failure and high patient satisfaction, just as among women without substance abuse histories.[73] Immediate post-placental intrauterine device (IUD) insertion is acceptable to women[74] and safe,[75] and eliminates the barriers related to the need to return to an outpatient setting for IUD insertion at six weeks postpartum.[76]

Transition to Primary Care

Access to primary care is important for all women and perhaps more crucial for women with physical and mental health issues related to past substance abuse.[35] Encouraging women to seek appropriate primary care, whether by continuing visits with the current provider or transitioning to another nonobstetric provider, is an important message after delivery or pregnancy loss or termination. Pregnancy often serves as an entry point to health care for women and the opportunity to engage women in comprehensive, ongoing care should not be lost. For obstetric providers who do not provide comprehensive primary care, developing a referral relationship with a clinician who can do so and who is able to demonstrate respect and compas-sion for women affected by substance abuse can facilitate a smooth transition of care.

SUMMARY

Optimal care of women with substance abuse disorders in pregnancy requires a multi-disciplinary approach (**Table 1**) that emphasizes respect, compassion, and flexibility. Pregnancy often serves as an opportunity for women to engage in healthy change.

Table 1	
Key aspects of care for pregnant women with substance use disorders	
Prenatal	
Pregnancy options counseling	Parenting, adoption, abortion
Substance abuse history	Substance(s), route, duration, withdrawal symptoms
Patient education	Effects of substances on pregnancy Postpartum contraception Breastfeeding Labor analgesia Preparation for parenting
Substance abuse counseling	Consideration for residential treatment
Harm reduction	Respectful, nonjudgmental approach Flexible scheduling Anticipate relapses
Opioid replacement therapy	Methadone or buprenorphine
Assessment and treatment of comorbidities	Medical: tobacco use, STIs, hepatitis C, dental disease Psychiatric: depression, bipolar disorder, anxiety, PTSD Environmental: intimate partner violence, homelessness, food insecurity
Fetal well-being	Serial fundal heights, selective use of ultrasound for growth and fetal surveillance
Intrapartum	
Opioid replacement therapy	Continue in labor Continue on day of scheduled cesarean section
Labor analgesia	Epidural is effective Parenteral pure opioid agonists are acceptable Avoid mixed agonist-antagonists in opioid-dependent women
Fetal heart rate monitoring	Avoid internal monitors in hepatitis C and HIV
Postpartum	
Postpartum pain management	Higher opioid dose requirements postoperatively in opioid-dependent women Can divide buprenorphine QID Appropriate NSAIDs and acetaminophen
Relapse prevention	Close follow-up Screen for depression Ask about drug cravings and relapse
Breastfeeding guidance	Stable patients on opioid replacement Hepatitis C acceptable (if no cracked/bleeding nipples) Contraindicated in active substance abuse and HIV
Contraceptive management	Sterilization if desired by patient Otherwise encourage long-acting reversible contraception Offer immediate post-placental IUD insertion
Transition to primary care	Pediatric developmental assessment and support Adult primary care

Although there are many challenges for clinicians and barriers to care for patients, successful treatment of substance abuse in pregnancy offers a chance to improve the lives of generations to come by helping women deliver and parent healthier children and by interrupting the legacy of addiction and family dysfunction inherited by so many women and their families.

REFERENCES

1. Substance Abuse and Mental Health Services Administration. Results from the 2012 national survey on drug use and health: summary of national findings. 2013. p. 22–4.
2. Patrick S, Shcumacher R, Bennyworth B, et al. Neonatal abstinence syndrome and associated health care expenditures: United states, 2000-2009. J Am Med Assoc 2012;307(18):E1.
3. Minnes S, Lang A, Singer L. Prenatal tobacco, marijuana, stimulant, and opiate exposure: outcomes and practice implications. Addict Sci Clin Pract 2011;6:57.
4. Morse B, Gehshan S, Hutchins E. Screening for substance abuse during pregnancy: improving care, improving health. U.S. Department of Health and Human Services. Health Resources and Services Administration. National Center for Education in Maternal and Child Health. 1997.
5. Lester BM, ElSohly M, Wright LL, et al. The maternal lifestyle study: drug use by meconium toxicology and maternal self-report. Pediatrics 2001;107(2):309.
6. Sokol RJ, Martier SS, Ager JW. The T-ACE questions: practical prenatal detection of risk-drinking. Am J Obstet Gynecol 1989;160(4):863–8 [discussion: 868–70].
7. Russell M. New assessment tools for risk drinking during pregnancy. Alcohol Health Res World 1994;18(1):55.
8. American College of Obstetricians and Gynecologists Committee on Ethics. At-risk drinking and ilicit drug use: ethical issues in obstetric and gynecologic practice. Obstet Gynecol 2008;112(6):1449.
9. Roberts S, Pies C. Complex calculations: how drug use during pregnancy becomes a barrier to prenatal care. Matern Child Health J 2011;15:333.
10. Bureau of Justice Statistics. Prisoners in 2012: Trends in admissions and releases, 1991-2012. 2013; NCJ 243920.
11. Ferszt G, Clarke J. Health care of pregnant women in U.S. state prisons. J Health Care Poor Underserved 2012;23(2):557.
12. Nunn A, Zaller N, Dickman S, et al. Methadone and buprenorphine prescribing and referral practices in US prison systems: results from a nationwide survey. Drug Alcohol Depend 2009;105:83.
13. Funai EF, White J, Lee MJ, et al. Compliance with prenatal care visits in substance users. J Matern Fetal Neonatal Med 2003;14(5):329.
14. Coleman-Cowger VH. Mental health treatment need among pregnant and postpartum women/girls entering substance abuse treatment. Psychol Addict Behav 2012;26(2):345–50.
15. Ordean A, Kahan M. Comprehensive treatment program for pregnant substance users in a family medicine clinic. Can Fam Physician 2011;57(11):e430–5.
16. Heil SH, Jones HE, Arria A, et al. Unintended pregnancy in opioid-abusing women. J Subst Abuse Treat 2011;40(2):199.
17. Marlatt GA. Harm reduction: come as you are. Addict Behav 1996;21(6):779.
18. Jones HE, Martin PR, Heil SH, et al. Treatment of opioid-dependent pregnant women: clinical and research issues. J Subst Abuse Treat 2008;35(3):245.
19. Pecoraro A, Ma M, Woody G. The science and practice of medication-assisted treatments for opioid dependence. Subst Use Misuse 2012;47:1026.
20. Bart G. Maintenance medication for opiate addiction: the foundation of recovery. J Addict Dis 2012;31(3):207.
21. Gibson A, Degenhardt L, Mattick R, et al. Exposure to opioid maintenance treatment reduces long-term mortality. Addiction 2008;103:462.

22. Wong S, Ordean A, Kahan M, Society of Obstetricians and Gynecologists of Canada. SOGC clinical practice guidelines: substance use in pregnancy: no. 256, April 2011. Int J Gynaecol Obstet 2011;114(2):190–202.
23. Doberczak T, Thornton J, Bernstein J, et al. Impact of maternal drug dependency on birth weight and head circumference of offspring. Am J Dis Child 1987;141(11):1163.
24. Hulse G, Milne E, English D, et al. The relationship between maternal use of heroin and methadone and infant birth weight. Addiction 1997;92(11):1571.
25. Dahan A. Opioid-induced respiratory effects: new data on buprenorphine. Palliat Med 2006;20(Suppl 1):s3.
26. Center for Substance Abuse Treatment. Medication-assisted treatment for opioid addiction in opioid treatment programs. 2005; Treatment Improvement Protocol Series 43. Report of the Substance Abuse and Mental Health Services Administration. HHS Publication No. (SMA) 12–4214.
27. Kraus ML, Alford DP, Kotz MM, et al. Statement of the american society of addiction medicine consensus panel on the use of buprenorphine in office-based treatment of opioid addiction. J Addict Med 2011;5(4):254–63.
28. Jones HE, Grady K, Malfi D, et al. Methadone maintenance vs. methadone taper during pregnancy: maternal and neonatal outcomes. Am J Addict 2008; 17:372.
29. Stewart RD, Nelson DB, Adhikari EH, et al. The obstetrical and neonatal impact of maternal opioid detoxification in pregnancy. Am J Obstet Gynecol 2013; 209(3):e1–5.
30. Yuan C, Foss JF, O'Connor M, et al. Gut motility and transit changes in patients receiving long-term methadone maintenance. J Clin Pharmacol 1998;38(10): 931–5.
31. Winstock AR, Lea T, Sheridan J. Patients' help-seeking behaviours for health problems associated with methadone and buprenorphine treatment. Drug Alcohol Rev 2008;27(4):393–7.
32. Hudak M, Tan R. Neonatal drug withdrawal. Pediatrics 2012;129:e540.
33. Jones HE, Kaltenbach K, Heil SH, et al. Neonatal abstinence syndrome after methadone or buprenorphine exposure. N Engl J Med 2010;363(24):2320–31.
34. Pearson FS, Prendergast ML, Podus D, et al. Meta-analyses of seven of the national institute on drug abuse's principles of drug addiction treatment. J Subst Abuse Treat 2012;43(1):1–11.
35. De Alba I, Samet JH, Saitz R. Burden of medical illness in drug- and alcohol-dependent persons without primary care. Am J Addict 2004;13(1):33–45.
36. Fan J, Hser YI, Herbeck D. Tooth retention, tooth loss and use of dental care among long-term narcotics abusers. Subst Abus 2006;27(1–2):25–32.
37. Rogers JM. Tobacco and pregnancy. Reprod Toxicol 2009;28(2):152–60.
38. Coleman T, Chamberlain C, Cooper S, et al. Efficacy and safety of nicotine replacement therapy for smoking cessation in pregnancy: systematic review and meta-analysis. Addiction 2011;106(1):52.
39. Haug NA, Svikis DS, Diclemente C. Motivational enhancement therapy for nicotine dependence in methadone-maintained pregnant women. Psychol Addict Behav 2004;18(3):289.
40. Chamberlain C, O'Mara-Eves A, Oliver S, et al. Psychosocial interventions for supporting women to stop smoking in pregnancy. Cochrane Database Syst Rev 2013;(10):CD001055.
41. Mehta G, Rothstein K. Health maintenance issues in cirrhosis. Med Clin North Am 2009;93(4):901.

42. American College of Obstetricians and Gynecologists Women's Health Care Physicians, Committee on Health Care for Underserved Women. Committee opinion no. 569: oral health care during pregnancy and through the lifespan. Obstet Gynecol 2013;122(2 Pt 1):417–22.

43. American College of Obstetricians and Gynecologists, Committee on Obstetric Practice. Committee opinion no. 453: screening for depression during and after pregnancy. Obstet Gynecol 2010;115(2 Pt 1):394–5.

44. Leddy MA, Lawrence H, Schulkin J. Obstetrician-gynecologists and women's mental health: findings of the collaborative ambulatory research network 2005-2009. Obstet Gynecol Surv 2011;66(5):316–23.

45. Helmbrecht GD, Thiagarajah S. Management of addiction disorders in pregnancy. J Addict Med 2008;2(1):1–16.

46. Festinger DS, Lamb RJ, Marlowe DB, et al. From telephone to office: intake attendance as a function of appointment delay. Addict Behav 2002;27(1): 131–7.

47. Kakko J, Heilig M, Sarman I. Buprenorphine and methadone treatment of opiate dependence during pregnancy: comparison of fetal growth and neonatal outcomes in two consecutive case series. Drug Alcohol Depend 2008;96(1–2): 69–78.

48. Ladhani NN, Shah PS, Murphy KE, Knowledge Synthesis Group on Determinants of Preterm/LBW Births. Prenatal amphetamine exposure and birth outcomes: a systematic review and metaanalysis. Am J Obstet Gynecol 2011; 205(3):219.e1–7.

49. Gouin K, Murphy K, Shah PS. Effects of cocaine use during pregnancy on low birthweight and preterm birth: systematic review and metaanalyses. Obstet Gynecol 2011;204(4):340.e1–12.

50. Ogunyemi D, Hernández-Loera GE. The impact of antenatal cocaine use on maternal characteristics and neonatal outcomes. J Matern Fetal Neonatal Med 2004;15(4):253–9.

51. Stewart JL, Meeker JE. Fetal and infant deaths associated with maternal methamphetamine abuse. J Anal Toxicol 1997;21(6):515–7.

52. American College of Obstetricians and Gynecologists Committee on Health Care for Underserved Women. Committee opinion no. 479: methamphetamine abuse in women of reproductive age. Obstet Gynecol 2011;117(3):751–5.

53. Appleyard K, Berlin LJ, Rosanbalm KD, et al. Preventing early child maltreatment: implications from a longitudinal study of maternal abuse history, substance use problems, and offspring victimization. Prev Sci 2011;12(2):139–49.

54. Suchman N, Pajulo M, Decoste C, et al. Parenting interventions for drug-dependent mothers and their young children: the case for an attachment-based approach. Fam Relat 2006;55(2):211–26.

55. Salisbury AL, Coyle MG, O'Grady KE, et al. Fetal assessment before and after dosing with buprenorphine or methadone. Addiction 2012;107(Suppl 1):36–44.

56. Cottrell EB, Chou R, Wasson N, et al. Reducing risk for mother-to-infant transmission of hepatitis C virus: a systematic review for the U.S. preventive services task force. Ann Intern Med 2013;158(2):109–13.

57. Maiques V, Garcia-Tejedor A, Perales A, et al. Intrapartum fetal invasive procedures and perinatal transmission of HIV. Eur J Obstet Gynecol Reprod Biol 1999; 87(1):63–7.

58. ACOG Committee on Health Care for Underserved Women, American Society of Addiction Medicine. ACOG committee opinion no. 524: opioid abuse, dependence, and addiction in pregnancy. Obstet Gynecol 2012;119(5):1070–6.

59. Meyer M, Wagner K, Benvenuto A, et al. Intrapartum and postpartum analgesia for women maintained on methadone during pregnancy. Obstet Gynecol 2007; 110(2 Pt 1):261–6.

60. Carroll IR, Angst MS, Clark JD. Management of perioperative pain in patients chronically consuming opioids. Reg Anesth Pain Med 2004;29(6):576–91.

61. Holbrook A, Kaltenbach K. Co-occurring psychiatric symptoms in opioid-dependent women: the prevalence of antenatal and postnatal depression. Am J Drug Alcohol Abuse 2012;38(6):575–9.

62. Chapman SL, Wu LT. Postpartum substance use and depressive symptoms: a review. Women Health 2013;53(5):479–503.

63. Academy of Breastfeeding Medicine Protocol Committee, Jansson LM. ABM clinical protocol #21: guidelines for breastfeeding and the drug-dependent woman. Breastfeed Med 2009;4(4):225–8.

64. Ilett KF, Hackett LP, Gower S, et al. Estimated dose exposure of the neonate to buprenorphine and its metabolite norbuprenorphine via breastmilk during maternal buprenorphine substitution treatment. Breastfeed Med 2012;7: 269–74.

65. Bogen DL, Perel JM, Helsel JC, et al. Estimated infant exposure to enantiomer-specific methadone levels in breastmilk. Breastfeed Med 2011;6(6):377–84.

66. Welle-Strand GK, Skurtveit S, Jansson LM, et al. Breastfeeding reduces the need for withdrawal treatment in opioid-exposed infants. Acta Paediatr 2013; 102(11):1060–6.

67. O'Connor AB, Collett A, Alto WA, et al. Breastfeeding rates and the relationship between breastfeeding and neonatal abstinence syndrome in women maintained on buprenorphine during pregnancy. J Midwifery Womens Health 2013;58(4):383–8.

68. Section on Breastfeeding. Breastfeeding and the use of human milk. Pediatrics 2012;129(3):e827–41.

69. Niccols A, Milligan K, Sword W, et al. Integrated programs for mothers with substance abuse issues: a systematic review of studies reporting on parenting outcomes. Harm Reduct J 2012;9:14.

70. Ordean A, Kahan M, Graves L, et al. Integrated care for pregnant women on methadone maintenance treatment: Canadian primary care cohort study. Can Fam Physician 2013;59(10):e462–9.

71. Blunt B. Supporting mothers in recovery: parenting classes. Neonatal Netw 2009;28(4):231–5.

72. Hernandez LE, Sappenfield WM, Goodman D, et al. Is effective contraceptive use conceived prenatally in florida? the association between prenatal contraceptive counseling and postpartum contraceptive use. Matern Child Health J 2012;16(2):423–9.

73. Espey E, Ogburn T. Long-acting reversible contraceptives: intrauterine devices and the contraceptive implant. Obstet Gynecol 2011;117(3):705–19.

74. Levi E, Cantillo E, Ades V, et al. Immediate postplacental IUD insertion at cesarean delivery: A prospective cohort study. Contraception 2012;86(2):102–5.

75. Kapp N, Curtis KM. Intrauterine device insertion during the postpartum period: A systematic review. Contraception 2009;80(4):327–36.

76. Ogburn JA, Espey E, Stonehocker J. Barriers to intrauterine device insertion in postpartum women. Contraception 2005;72(6):426–9.

Teratogenic Risks from Exposure to Illicit Drugs

Bradley D. Holbrook, MD*, William F. Rayburn, MD, MBA

KEYWORDS

- Addiction • Fetal effects • Illicit drug use • Teratogenic risk
- Pregnancy complications

KEY POINTS

- This article presents issues pertaining to limitations with reports about fetal risks and describes current information in humans about fetal effects for specific illicit drugs.
- Associating illicit drug use with eventual pregnancy outcome is difficult. Concurrent use with multiple substances is frequent, and many users are economically disadvantaged, which contributes to unfavorable perinatal outcomes.
- Teratogenic effects may be manifested not only as an intrauterine demise or dysmorphism, but also as growth restriction or behavioral changes.
- Except for maternal alcohol exposure, no birth defect syndrome has been described for specific illicit substances or prescription drugs of abuse.

INTRODUCTION

Substance use is prevalent in the United States, especially in the reproductive-age population. The 2012 National Survey on Drug Use and Health indicated that 14.7% of the US population aged 12 or older used an illicit drug and 4.9% used prescription-type pain relievers for nonmedical reasons in the past year.[1] Furthermore, 9% of this population had some form of substance use disorder. Cigarette and binge alcohol use (five or more drinks on at least one occasion in past 30 days) involved 24.1% and 23.2% of the population, respectively.

Chronic substance use may affect menstrual cycles and semen analysis, but these effects are generally reversible with discontinuation of the drug.[2–5] For this reason, reproductive-age women with addiction disorders may still conceive at any time. Delivery of a drug or chemical by the sperm to the oocyte may be associated with

The authors have nothing to disclose.

Division of Maternal-Fetal Medicine, Department of Obstetrics and Gynecology, University of New Mexico School of Medicine, MSC10 5580, 1 University of New Mexico, Albuquerque, NM 87131–0001, USA

* Corresponding author.

E-mail address: BHolbrook@salud.unm.edu

Obstet Gynecol Clin N Am 41 (2014) 229–239

http://dx.doi.org/10.1016/j.ogc.2014.02.008

0889-8545/14/$ – see front matter © 2014 Elsevier Inc. All rights reserved.

developmental toxicity, although less is understood and toxicity has not been well-demonstrated in humans.

Illicit drugs include cannabis, stimulants, cocaine (including crack), heroin, hallucinogens, inhalants, or prescription-type psychotherapeutics used nonmedically. According to the 2012 National Survey on Drug Use and Health, an estimated 4.4% of pregnant women reported illicit drug use in the past 30 days.[1] A second study showed that whereas 0.1% of pregnant women were estimated to have used heroin in the past 30 days, 1% of pregnant women reported nonmedical use of an opioid-containing pain medication.[6] Even though a reduction in substance use may occur during pregnancy, some women may not alter their drug use patterns until at least pregnancy is confirmed. For these reasons, a large number of fetuses are exposed to illicit substances, including during critical stages of organogenesis.

Associating illicit drug use with eventual pregnancy outcome is difficult, because concurrent use of multiple substances is frequent and many users are members of economically disadvantaged segments of society in which unfavorable perinatal outcomes are more common. It is also difficult to follow infant outcomes in such pregnancies and to analyze research data. This article presents issues pertaining to limitations with published investigations about fetal risks and describes the most current information in humans about fetal effects from specific illicit substances (**Table 1**).

LIMITATIONS WITH INVESTIGATIONS ABOUT FETAL RISKS

Difficulties in accurately monitoring dose and exposure of a substance continue to undermine the strength of many observations regarding adverse perinatal effects. Illicit drugs and prescription medications for recreational reasons may be intentionally or inadvertently taken at potentially toxic doses. An accurate evaluation of dosage and the exact period of exposure are often not possible. Addiction or the recreational use of illicit substances may lead to the intake of these drugs in large and uncontrolled doses. For example, when amphetamine use has been studied among addicted mothers, it has been difficult to identify which adverse effects may have resulted from these drugs or the simultaneous use of other substances (eg, ethanol), and poor maternal nutrition, hygiene, and attendance at prenatal visits.

Any illicit drug unbound to proteins can freely pass from the maternal compartment, across the placenta, and into the fetal compartment. Concentrations in the fetal serum can be the same or even higher than in the mother. Little doubt exists that passage of the drug or metabolite into the fetal central nervous system is unimpeded. Effects on the developing embryo and fetus depend on gestational timing, extent of drug distribution, uteroplacental perfusion, and drug or metabolite amount.

Teratogenic effects may be manifested not only as an intrauterine demise or dysmorphism, but also as growth restriction or behavioral changes. Although an association between a substance and an anomaly (eg, midline facial defects) may be suggested with a particular genetic susceptibility, subsequent epidemiologic studies often do not ascribe any substance exposure with an increase in human malformations. It is also not possible to conclude in human beings that heritable birth defects are increased after exposure to a certain drug or chemical.

Small population sizes and unblinded evaluations of drug-exposed newborns raise questions about the significance of any teratogenic observations. Other causes for adverse pregnancy outcome may also exist within drug-abusing populations. Impurity of most illicit drugs and the common practice of using multiple substances either combined or at separate times make it difficult to ascribe specific fetal effects to a certain compound.

Table 1
Suspected effects described in humans after exposure to illicit drugs during pregnancy

Illicit Drug	Effects on Mother/ Pregnancy	Potential Structural Effects	Neurobehavioral Effects
Cannabis	Shorter gestation Lower birth weight	None specific	Impaired executive function
Opioids	Preterm delivery PPROM Meconium-stained amniotic fluid IUGR Chorioamnionitis Fetal death	Congenital heart defects Neural tube defect	Neonatal abstinence syndrome Aggressiveness Impulsiveness Increased temper Poorer self-confidence Impaired memory Impaired perception
Cocaine	Preterm delivery Placental abruption Uterine rupture Fetal death IUGR	Necrotizing enterocolitis Disagreement regarding structural defects	Impaired language development Attention deficits in males Inhibition deficits in males
Amphetamines	Maternal psychiatric diagnosis	Oral clefts Smaller head circumference Shorter length Disagreement regarding other structural defects	Increased emotional reactivity Depression Anxiety ADHD Externalizing behavior Aggressiveness
Hallucinogens	No data	PCP: Microcephaly Abnormal facies Intracranial abnormalities Respiratory anomalies Cardiovascular defects Urinary tract anomalies Musculoskeletal abnormalities LSD: Limb defects Ocular abnormalities MDMA: Congenital heart disease Musculoskeletal abnormalities Peyote: No data	PCP: Attachment disorder LSD: No data MDMA: Impaired motor abilities at 4 mo Peyote: No data
Inhalants	Maternal electrolyte abnormalities Maternal arrhythmias Maternal RTA IUGR Preterm labor	Microcephaly Craniofacial abnormalities similar to those seen in fetal alcohol syndrome	Developmental delay Growth impairment Attention deficits Language deficits Cerebellar dysfunction

Abbreviations: ADHD, attention-deficit/hyperactivity disorder; IUGR, intrauterine growth restriction; LSD, lysergic acid diethylamide; MDMA, 3,4-methylenedioxymethamphetamine (ecstasy); PCP, phencyclidine; PPROM, preterm premature rupture of membranes; RTA, renal tubular acidosis.

Besides maternal alcohol, a birth defect syndrome has not been described for illicit substances or prescription drugs of abuse. The broad range of the described defects makes definition of a single syndrome difficult. Many controlled studies have observed an increase in birth defects with certain substances during human pregnancy. The lack of uniformity among the defects, insufficient number of study cases, and failure to use a comparable group of non–drug-using women as control subjects cast doubt on the relative risks. The inconsistency in these retrospective associations, along with criticisms about potential bias in data collection, makes it unjustified to consider a given illicit drug as causing these malformations. It has been recently demonstrated, however, that use of tobacco (including secondhand smoke exposure) or any illicit drug leads to an increased risk of stillbirth.[7]

Measuring the in utero effect of alcohol and substance exposure on infant and child development also presents many challenges. Although animal studies indicate that alcohol and drugs reduce the density of cortical neurons and change dendritic connections, their significance in human development is unclear.[8] Altered fetal behaviors are usually insidious, variable, and not easily recognized. Measureable effects during lengthy periods of development can less precisely implicate a prior drug exposure. Social, cultural, environmental, and genetic factors are influential, so evidence of altered behavior or impaired development in previously exposed children may not only measure teratogenic effects of substances but also parental influences on behavior.

Risks from exposure to illicit drugs during breastfeeding are less of an issue. A substance and its active metabolites enter breast milk in undetermined quantities and are usually absorbed in small amounts by the neonate. Accumulated substances in exposed infants can contribute to poor suckling, irritability, or somnolence. For this reason, repeated use of psychotherapeutic drugs or illicit substances by nursing mothers is not recommended by the American Academy of Pediatrics.[9]

EFFECTS FROM SPECIFIC ILLICIT DRUGS
Cannabis

Marijuana smoke contains many compounds. The most active and most well-studied of these is Δ9-tetrahydrocannabinol, which binds to the cannabinoid receptors of the central nervous system. Intoxication leads to an elevated heart rate, a feeling of euphoria, decreased alertness, decrease in motor stability, congestion, and increased appetite, although the mechanism through which it achieves these is not clear.[10]

Numerous published studies and case reports describe no patterns between maternal cannabis use and malformations. There is an increased incidence of low birth weight among neonates born to mothers who used marijuana during pregnancy.[11] This may relate to smoking marijuana more than five times per week being associated with a slightly shortened gestation by 0.8 weeks.[11,12]

Unlike most other substances of abuse, marijuana has been extensively studied in a longitudinal manner to evaluate long-term neurobehavioral outcomes. The Ottawa Prenatal Prospective study followed a long-term cohort of children exposed in utero to marijuana. In the toddler stage, there was no evidence of impaired growth or behavior. However, after age 3, there are notable differences in executive function (behaviors associated with impulsivity, attention, and problem solving).[13] It is speculated that cannabinoids may differentially impact the developing frontal lobe.

Opioids

Opioids bind to opioid receptors of the central nervous system, leading to a decreased sensation of pain without loss of consciousness, and often accompanied by a feeling of euphoria. Physiologic effects of these drugs include decreased sympathetic tone and histamine release, which lead to respiratory depression, sedation, decreased gastrointestinal motility, itching, miosis, and urinary retention.[14,15]

Opioid use during pregnancy has been associated with increased complications, such as preterm delivery,[16] preterm premature rupture of membranes, meconium-stained amniotic fluid, intrauterine growth restriction, chorioamnionitis, and perinatal death.[16–18] Fetuses exposed to opioids in utero are more likely than their peers to have any birth defect. A 2011 analysis of data in the National Birth Defects Prevention Study reported statistically significant associations between the use of opioid medications in the interval from 1 month before to 3 months after conception and the following defects: conoventricular septal defects (odds ratio [OR], 2.7; 95% confidence interval [CI], 1.1–6.3), atrioventricular septal defects (OR, 2.0; 95% CI, 1.2–3.6), hypoplastic left heart syndrome (OR, 2.4; 95% CI, 1.4–4.1), spina bifida (OR, 2.0; 95% CI, 1.3–3.2), and gastroschisis (OR, 1.8; 95% CI, 1.1–2.9).[19] The authors noted the limitations of their data, which relied on maternal recall of drugs used and did not take into account dosage or the use of combination products. No specific pattern of birth defects has been identified, however, raising the question as to whether there are confounding variables that were not controlled in those studies.[17,18]

Neonatal abstinence syndrome (NAS) is a well-described sequelae of neonates exposed to opioids in utero. Withdrawal causes autonomic hyperactivity, characterized by fever, irritability, hypertonia, diarrhea, feeding dysfunction, and sleep disturbances.[20] The severity of NAS does not seem to vary with different maternal doses of methadone.[21] More is written about this syndrome and its management elsewhere in this issue.

Methadone and buprenorphine are used as alternatives to heroin or other opioid use to decrease associated high-risk maternal behaviors. These maintenance medications have not been definitively shown to have any greater or lesser effect than heroin on the developing fetus, nor do they prevent NAS. Because of its longer half-life, methadone may cause more severe or prolonged NAS compared with buprenorphine.[22]

Throughout childhood, children chronically exposed to opioids in utero have been shown to have slight differences from their nonexposed peers of similar socioeconomic backgrounds. Exposed children showed increased episodes of temper, impulsiveness, and aggressiveness, and poorer self-confidence.[23] Tests of memory and perception revealed impaired abilities in these realms.[23] Body measurements also revealed lower weight and smaller head circumference.[24]

The American Academy of Pediatrics recommends against the use of heroin or other nonprescription opioids by breastfeeding mothers.[9] This contrasts with mothers maintained on methadone or buprenorphine who are encouraged to breastfeed because this has led to less severe NAS symptoms in multiple studies.[24,25] Opioids are commonly used for pain control after cesarean deliveries and this is not a contraindication to breastfeeding.[9] However, there is a recent case of neonatal death from morphine overdose in a nursing infant whose mother was taking codeine and later found to be a rapid metabolizer of codeine into morphine.[26] This has led the Food and Drug Administration to advise against the use of codeine in nursing mothers, unless the mother is known to not metabolize codeine rapidly.[27]

Cocaine

Cocaine blocks reuptake of catecholamines and serotonin and enhances presynaptic release of these same substances from peripheral nerve terminals. Vasoconstriction and transient hypertension result from systemic sympathetic effects. In the limbic system, there is an increased release of excitatory amino acids glutamate and aspartate.

Cocaine also has a local anesthetic effect because of its blockade of sodium channels.[28] These effects can cause specific problems during pregnancy because this vasoconstriction may lead to decreased placental perfusion.[29]

Cocaine has been linked to several fetal anomalies including craniofacial abnormalities, limb deformities, and urinary tract anomalies. However, more recent analyses shed doubt on those findings. A large, prospective multisite study examining 717 cocaine-exposed pregnancies indicated that structural abnormalities are no higher in cocaine-exposed infants than control subjects.[30]

Fetal growth can be impaired, with an increased incidence of intrauterine growth restriction among these fetuses.[30,31] Longitudinal studies have revealed that these children do tend to catch up to a normal weight range by 6.5 and 13 months of life, although they may be slightly shorter than their peers. It is unclear whether this short stature is caused by cocaine or a confounder more likely caused by concomitant alcohol use.[32]

Pregnancies exposed to cocaine have an increased incidence of preterm delivery[31] and placental abruption[33]; cases of uterine rupture[34] and fetal death[35] associated with maternal cocaine use also have been reported. Necrotizing enterocolitis seems to be increased among neonates exposed to cocaine in utero.[36] There is disagreement regarding whether the rate of sudden infant death syndrome is also increased. A meta-analysis concluded that there is an increased risk of sudden infant death syndrome in any infant exposed to drugs in utero, but no increased risk was found specifically for cocaine use alone.[37]

Cocaine also affects fetal and postnatal behavior. Symptoms of acute fetal intoxication and withdrawal have been observed sonographically.[38] With chronic use, ultrasound findings of abnormal fetal behavioral state organization and regulation were viewed, which correlated with similar abnormal behaviors viewed in the neonatal period.[38] After birth, language development is impaired.[39] Males (but not females) exposed to cocaine have been shown to have deficits with attention and inhibition.[40]

Amphetamines

Amphetamines act as indirect sympathomimetics by increasing the concentration of catecholamines at the postsynaptic terminal through blockade of reuptake (similar to cocaine), and increasing release of dopamine and norepinephrine. These lead to systemic sympathetic effects, such as increased heart rate, cardiac output, and blood pressure; dilated pupils; and bronchodilation.[41]

Retrospective studies and case reports have suggested that methamphetamine use is associated with pregnancy complications, such as hypertensive disease, postpartum hemorrhage, and retained placenta. However, a more recent prospective study seems to disprove these findings, revealing an absence of serious maternal complications with the exception of maternal psychiatric disorders.[42] Case reports have linked maternal amphetamine use with congenital heart disease, biliary atresia, and gastroschisis. A prospective study did not confirm any of these associations, however, but did find an increased incidence of oral clefts.[43] Infants exposed to methamphetamines do have a smaller head circumference and shorter length than their peers.[42] Neonates exposed to amphetamines in utero exhibited poor suck, increased jitteriness, and autonomic stress, and were more likely to be admitted to the neonatal intensive care unit after birth.[42]

Throughout childhood, these children often suffer from several behavioral and developmental issues. However, these do not seem directly the result of methamphetamine exposure. A study that compared methamphetamine-exposed children raised in normal versus high-risk environments found that neurobehavioral deficits in these children at 3 years of age could be attributed to their environment.[44] When data from these same study subjects were examined at both 3 and 5 years of age and compared with control subjects, significant deficits were noted. There was an increase in emotional reactivity and anxiety and depression at both 3 and 5 years. At 5 years only, an increase in attention-deficit/hyperactivity disorder was noted, as was an increase in externalizing and aggressive behavior. These findings were more marked for boys than girls, and were also more severe in the offspring of mothers with heavy methamphetamine use, defined as more than three times per week.[45]

Hallucinogens

Hallucinogens are a diverse class of compounds. The pharmacology of these substances is quite varied, but all seem to act through serotonin pathways in the central nervous system.[46] Of these multiple compounds, the most commonly abused are phencyclidine, lysergic acid diethylamide (LSD), and 3,4-methylenedioxymethamphetamine (MDMA, commonly known as "ecstasy"). Native Americans are known to smoke buttons from the peyote cactus in religious ceremonies.[47] The active substance in peyote is mescaline, which is also a hallucinogen.

Literature evaluating the outcomes of fetuses exposed to hallucinogens is sparse. Nearly all reported experiences are published cases and, thus, quite limited. Phencyclidine use has been linked to birth defects, such as microcephaly[48] and abnormal facies.[49] Another case report found significant intracranial abnormalities and defects of the cardiovascular, respiratory, urinary, and musculoskeletal systems with subsequent neonatal death.[50] After delivery, these infants may display increased tone and jitteriness, and lethargy.[49] Sleep disturbances and abnormal temperament have also been described.[51] Through the first year of life, an attachment disorder was described, but there is no evidence of other behavioral deficits.[51]

Case reports exist of prenatal LSD exposure leading to defects, such as limb defects and eye abnormalities.[52,53] There are no published studies or case reports evaluating neurobehavioral outcomes in children exposed to LSD in utero.

There are limited data regarding MDMA ("ecstasy") use in pregnancy. One study demonstrated an increased risk of birth defects, most notably congenital heart disease and musculoskeletal abnormalities.[54] Another study of infants exposed to MDMA in utero described impaired motor abilities at 4 months but no other neurobehavioral defecits.[55]

There are no data regarding the effects of peyote use on human pregnancies.

Inhalants

Inhalants represent a diverse group of compounds that are inhaled to achieve intoxicating properties. These include solvents, such as toluene; fuels; anesthetics; nitrous oxide; and alkyl nitrites. Although these substances differ significantly, their pharmacologic and behavioral effects are quite similar and the effect is to produce an alcohol-like intoxication, characterized by euphoria, slurred speech, dizziness, incoordination, involuntary eye movement, slowed thinking, and lethargy.[56,57] The mechanism by which these physiologic effects is achieved is unknown. Although some may be exposed to these compounds in the workplace, concentrations to which abusers are exposed are approximately 50 times greater than the maximum allowed in the workplace.[58] Toluene is the most well-studied of these compounds and is found in many glues and other industrial chemicals that are abused as inhalants.

Medical complications seen in abusers of these substances include electrolyte disturbances, cardiac arrhythmias, and renal tubular acidosis.[59] Pregnancy is often complicated by preterm labor and intrauterine growth restriction; in one study of toluene-exposed pregnancies, these were observed in 42% and 52% of cases, respectively.[60]

Many structural defects have been noted in fetuses exposed to inhalants. Toluene has risk of microcephaly as high as 32% to 33%.[60,61] Also observed are other craniofacial abnormalities similar to those seen in fetal alcohol syndrome: narrow bifrontal diameter, hypoplastic midface, short palpebral fissures, wide nasal bridge, blunt fingertips, and abnormal palmar creases; these have been commonly seen in infants exposed to inhalants in the absence of alcohol exposure.[60]

Unfortunately, children exposed to toluene in utero exhibit significant long-term functional and neurobehavioral deficits. One report indicated that as many as 38% of affected children have some developmental delay.[60] Microcephaly is common. Overall growth can be impaired[60] even after birth as described in six of eight toluene-exposed children who were born with a normal head circumference.[61] Attention and language deficits are common.[59] Central nervous system impairment, including cerebellar dysfunction, has also been noted.[59]

SUMMARY

Pregnant women including those with addictive disorders are commonly concerned about health issues affecting their unborn babies and themselves. Counseling about harmful effects from in utero exposure to a specific illicit or prescription drug is often limited and with usually no defined congenital anomalies or long-term behavior patterns. Fetal ultrasound imaging for anatomy and growth is essential early and repeatedly during pregnancy, although most infants appear healthy at birth and appropriately sized with no birth defects. Many women with a recent history of substance abuse seek prenatal care but do not desire specialized clinics for addiction. Benefits from attending such specialized settings can be offset by difficulty with accessibility. Comprehensive care by qualified practitioners and treatment of alcohol and other drug addictions remain essential for women on the road to recovery and the welfare of their fetus. Regardless of the site of prenatal care, long-term provision of services (nutrition, counseling, social) is vital to fetal and newborn well-being. Continuity of care requires collaboration and cooperation among many community-based services, ranging from agencies that offer safe housing and programs that stress parenting education; encourage responsible breastfeeding; and address issues of domestic violence, abuse, and victimization. With the help of family and peers, these services give the mother the best chance of providing a drug-free environment for growth and development of their fetus or newborn infant. Furthermore, nonpunitive services can better identify and reduce behaviors in mothers whose attention to the infant and other children is reduced, thereby possibly improving on their child's development.

REFERENCES

1. Substance Abuse and Mental Health Services Administration. Results from the 2012 National Survey on Drug Use and Health: summary of national findings. NSDUH SeriesH-41, HHS Publication No. (SMA) 11–4658. Rockville (MD): SAHMSA; 2011. Available at: http://www.nas.samhsa.gov/NSDUH/2k10NSDUH/2k12Results.pdf. Accessed November 18, 2013.
2. Hugues JN, Coste T, Perret G. Hypothalamo-pituitary ovarian function in thirty-one women with chronic alcoholism. Clin Endocrinol 1980;12(6):543–51.
3. Hill M, Popov P, Havlikova H. Reinstatement of serum pregnanolone isomers and progesterone during alcohol detoxification therapy in premenopausal women. Alcohol Clin Exp Res 2005;29(6):1010–7.

4. Ragni G, De Lauretis L, Bestetti O, et al. Gonadal function in male heroin and methadone addicts. Int J Androl 1988;11(2):93–100.
5. Barazani Y, Katz BF, Nagler HM, et al. Lifestyle, environment, and male reproductive health. Urol Clin North Am 2014;41(1):55–66.
6. Azadi A, Dildy GA 3rd. Universal screening for substance abuse at the time of parturition. Am J Obstet Gynecol 2008;198:e30–2.
7. Varner MW, Silver RM, Rowland Hogue CJ, et al. Association between stillbirth and illicit drug use and smoking during pregnancy. Obstet Gynecol 2014; 123(1):113–25.
8. Kranzler H, Amin H, Lowe V, et al. Pharmacologic treatments for drug and alcohol dependence. Psychiatr Clin North Am 1999;22:202–39.
9. American Academy of Pediatrics Committee on Drugs. Transfer of drugs and other chemicals into human milk. Pediatrics 2001;108:776–89.
10. Borgelt LM, Franson KL, Nussbaum AM, et al. The pharmacologic and clinical effects of medical cannabis. Pharmacotherapy 2013;33(2):195–209.
11. Hingson R, Alpert JJ, Day N, et al. Effects of maternal drinking and marijuana use on fetal growth and development. Pediatrics 1982;70(4):539–46.
12. Fried PA, Watkinson B, Willan A. Marijuana use during pregnancy and decreased length of gestation. Am J Obstet Gynecol 1984;150(1):23–7.
13. Fried PA, Smith AM. A literature review of the consequences of prenatal marihuana exposure. An emerging theme of a deficiency in aspects of executive function. Neurotoxicol Teratol 2001;23(1):1–11.
14. Trescot AM, Datta S, Lee M. Opioid pharmacology. Pain Physician 2008;11: S133–53.
15. Yip L, Megarbane B, Borron SW. Opioids. In: Shannon MW, Borron SW, Burns MJ, editors. Haddad and Winchester's clinical management of poisoning and drug overdose. 4th edition. Philadelphia: Saunders/Elsevier; 2007. p. 637–8.
16. Fajemirokun-Odudeyi O, Sinha C, Tutty S, et al. Pregnancy outcome in women who use opiates. Eur J Obstet Gynecol Reprod Biol 2006;126(2):170–5.
17. Ostrea EM, Chavez CJ. Perinatal problems (excluding neonatal withdrawal) in maternal drug addiction: a study of 830 cases. J Pediatr 1979;94(2):292–5.
18. Naeye RL, Blanc W, Leblanc W, et al. Fetal complications of maternal heroin addiction: abnormal growth, infections, and episodes of stress. J Pediatr 1973;83(6):1055–61.
19. Broussard CS, Rasmussen SA, Reefhuis J, et al, National Birth Defects Prevention Study. Maternal treatment with opioid analgesics and risk for birth defects. Am J Obstet Gynecol 2011;204(4):314.e1–11.
20. Oei J, Lui K. Management of the newborn affected by maternal opiates and other drugs of dependency. J Paediatr Child Health 2007;43:9–18.
21. Berghella V, Lim PJ, Hill MK, et al. Maternal methadone dose and neonatal withdrawal. Obstet Gynecol 2003;101(5 Pt 2):1060–2.
22. Gaalema DE, Scott TL, Heil SH, et al. Differences in the profile of neonatal abstinence syndrome signs in methadone- versus buprenorphine-exposed neonates. Addiction 2012;107(Suppl 1):53–62.
23. Wilson GS, McCreary R, Kean J, et al. The development of preschool children of heroin-addicted mothers: a controlled study. Pediatrics 1979;63(1): 135–41.
24. Abdel-Latif ME, Pinner J, Clews S, et al. Effects of breast milk on the severity and outcome of neonatal abstinence syndrome among infants of drug-dependent mothers. Pediatrics 2006;117(6):e1163–9.

25. McQueen KA, Murphy-Oikonen J, Gerlach K, et al. The impact of infant feeding method on neonatal abstinence scores of methadone-exposed infants. Adv Neonatal Care 2011;11(4):282–90.
26. Koren G, Cairns J, Chitayat D, et al. Pharmacogenetics of morphine poisoning in a breastfed neonate of a codeine-prescribed mother. Lancet 2006;368(9536): 704.
27. United States Food and Drug Administration. FDA warning on codeine use by nursing mothers. Silver Spring (MD): United States Food and Drug Administration; 2007. Available at: http://www.fda.gov/NewsEvents/Newsroom/Press Announcements/2007/ucm108968.htm. Accessed December 21, 2013.
28. Albertson TE, Chan A, Tharratt RS. Cocaine. In: Shannon MW, Borron SW, Burns MJ, editors. Haddad and Winchester's clinical management of poisoning and drug overdose. 4th edition. Philadelphia: Saunders/Elsevier; 2007. p. 756–7.
29. Woods JR Jr, Plessinger MA, Clark KE. Effect of cocaine on uterine blood flow and fetal oxygenation. JAMA 1987;257(7):957–61.
30. Bauer CR, Langer JC, Shankaran S, et al. Acute neonatal effects of cocaine exposure during pregnancy. Arch Pediatr Adolesc Med 2005;159(9):824–34.
31. Gouin K, Murphy K, Shah PS. Effects of cocaine use during pregnancy on low birthweight and preterm birth: systematic review and metaanalyses. Am J Obstet Gynecol 2011;204(4):340.e1–2.
32. Jacobson JL, Jacobson SW, Sokol RJ. Effects of prenatal exposure to alcohol, smoking, and illicit drugs on postpartum somatic growth. Alcohol Clin Exp Res 1994;18(2):317–23.
33. Dombrowski MP, Wolfe HM, Welch RA, et al. Cocaine abuse is associated with abruptio placentae and decreased birth weight, but not shorter labor. Obstet Gynecol 1991;77:139–41.
34. Gonsoulin W, Borge D, Moise KJ. Rupture of unscarred uterus in primigravid woman in association with cocaine abuse. Am J Obstet Gynecol 1990;163: 526–7.
35. Gratacos E, Torres PJ, Antolin E. Use of cocaine during pregnancy. N Engl J Med 1993;329:667.
36. Czyrko C, Del Pin CA, O'Neill JA, et al. Maternal cocaine abuse and necrotizing enterocolitis: outcome and survival. J Pediatr Surg 1991;26(4):414–21.
37. Fares I, McCulloch KM, Raju TN. Intrauterine cocaine exposure and the risk for sudden infant death syndrome: a meta-analysis. J Perinatol 1997;17(3):179–82.
38. Hume RF, O'Donnell KJ, Stanger CL, et al. In utero cocaine exposure: observations of fetal behavioral state may predict neonatal outcome. Am J Obstet Gynecol 1989;161(3):685–90.
39. Bandstra ES, Marrow CE, Accornero VH, et al. Estimated effects of in utero cocaine exposure on language development through early adolescence. Neurotoxicol Teratol 2011;33(1):25–35.
40. Carmody DP, Bennett DS, Lewis M. The effects of prenatal cocaine exposure and gender on inhibitory control and attention. Neurotoxicol Teratol 2011; 33(1):61–8.
41. Albertson TE, Kenyon NJ, Morrissey B. Amphetamines and derivatives. In: Shannon MW, Borron SW, Burns MJ, editors. Haddad and Winchester's clinical management of poisoning and drug overdose. 4th edition. Philadelphia: Saunders/Elsevier; 2007. p. 783.
42. Shah R, Diaz SD, Arria A, et al. Prenatal methamphetamine exposure and short-term maternal and infant medical outcomes. Am J Perinatol 2012;29(5):391–400.

43. Milkovich L, van der Berg BJ. Effects of antenatal exposure to anorectic drugs. Am J Obstet Gynecol 1977;129(6):637–42.
44. Derauf C, LaGasse L, Smith L, et al. Infant temperament and high-risk environment relate to behavior problems and language in toddlers. J Dev Behav Pediatr 2011;32(2):125–35.
45. LaGasse LL, Derauf C, Smith LM, et al. Prenatal methamphetamine exposure and childhood behavior problems at 3 and 5 years of age. Pediatrics 2012; 129(4):681–8.
46. Traub SJ. Hallucinogens. In: Shannon MW, Borron SW, Burns MJ, editors. Haddad and Winchester's clinical management of poisoning and drug overdose. 4th edition. Philadelphia: Saunders/Elsevier; 2007. p. 796–7.
47. Fickenscher A, Novins DK, Manson SM. Illicit peyote use among American Indian adolescents in substance abuse treatment: a preliminary investigation. Subst Use Misuse 2006;41(8):1139–54.
48. Strauss AA, Modaniou HD, Bosu SK. Neonatal manifestations of maternal phencyclidine (PCP) abuse. Pediatrics 1981;68(4):550–2.
49. Golden NL, Sokol RJ, Rubin IL. Angel dust: possible effects on the fetus. Pediatrics 1990;65(1):18–20.
50. Michaud J, Mizrahi EM, Ulrick H. Agenesis of the vermis with fusion of the cerebellar hemispheres, septo-optic dysplasia and associated anomalies: report of a case. Acta Neuropathol 1982;56(3):161–6.
51. Wachsman L, Schuetz S, Chan LS, et al. What happens to babies exposed to phencyclidine (PCP) in utero? Am J Drug Alcohol Abuse 1989;15(1):31–9.
52. Apple DJ, Bennett TO. Multiple systemic and ocular malformation associated with maternal LSD usage. Arch Ophthalmol 1974;92(4):301–3.
53. Chan CC, Fishman M, Egbert PR. Multiple ocular anomalies associated with maternal LSD ingestion. Arch Ophthalmol 1978;96(2):282–4.
54. McElhatton PR, Bateman DN, Evans C, et al. Congenital anomalies after prenatal ecstasy exposure. Lancet 1999;354(9188):1441–2.
55. Singer LT, Moore DG, Fulton S, et al. Neurobehavioral outcomes of infants exposed to MDMA (ecstasy) and other recreational drugs during pregnancy. Neurotoxicol Teratol 2012;34(3):303–10.
56. Jones HE, Balster RL. Inhalant abuse in pregnancy. Obstet Gynecol Clin North Am 1998;25(1):153–67.
57. Howard MO, Bowen SE, Garland EL, et al. Inhalant use and inhalant use disorders in the United States. Addict Sci Clin Pract 2011;6(1):18–31.
58. Mirkin DB. Benzene and related aromatic hydrocarbons. In: Shannon MW, Borron SW, Burns MJ, editors. Haddad and Winchester's clinical management of poisoning and drug overdose. 4th edition. Philadelphia: Saunders/Elsevier; 2007. p. 1370–4.
59. Hannigan JH, Bowen SE. Reproductive toxicology and teratology of abused toluene. Syst Biol Reprod Med 2010;56(2):184–200.
60. Arnold GL, Kirby RS, Langendoerfer S, et al. Toluene embryopathy: clinical delineation and developmental follow-up. Pediatrics 1994;93(2):216–20.
61. Pearson MA, Hoyme HE, Seaver LH, et al. Toluene embryopathy: delineation of the phenotype and comparison with fetal alcohol syndrome. Pediatrics 1994; 93(2):211–5.

Buprenorphine and Methadone for Opioid Addiction During Pregnancy

Ellen L. Mozurkewich, MD, MS*, William F. Rayburn, MD, MBA

KEYWORDS

- Buprenorphine • Methadone • Pregnancy opioid addiction • Neonatal • Abstinence

KEY POINTS

- Opioid substitution therapy with methadone or buprenorphine during and after pregnancy, and postpartum, improves maternal and neonatal outcomes.
- It is expected that the physiologic changes of pregnancy, such as increases in maternal weight, intravascular volume, and renal elimination of drugs will necessitate increased dosage of opioid substitution medications during the second and third trimesters.
- Methadone therapy may be associated with higher treatment satisfaction and treatment retention in comparison with buprenorphine therapy.
- The only well-recognized adverse effect of opioid substitution therapy is the neonatal abstinence syndrome, which is common but not dose dependent. Compared with methadone therapy, buprenorphine therapy reduces duration and severity of neonatal abstinence syndrome.

INTRODUCTION

About 4% of pregnant women in the United States report current illicit drug use.[1] Opioid use during pregnancy has been reported to range between 1% and 21%.[1] Buprenorphine and methadone are opioid-receptor agonists used as opioid substitution therapy to limit the detrimental effects of illicit opioid use.[2] Opioid substitution therapy with buprenorphine or methadone is used during pregnancy to limit the exposure of the fetus to cycles of opioid withdrawal and reduce risk of infectious comorbidities of illicit opioid use.[1,2]

Most authorities do not recommend detoxification to abstinence-based recovery during pregnancy because of theoretical risks to the fetus posed by intrauterine opioid

The authors have nothing to disclose.
Division of Maternal Fetal Medicine, Department of Obstetrics and Gynecology, University of New Mexico School of Medicine, MSC 10 5580, 1 University of New Mexico, Albuquerque, NM 87131, USA
* Corresponding author.
E-mail address: emozurkewich@salud.unm.edu

Obstet Gynecol Clin N Am 41 (2014) 241–253
http://dx.doi.org/10.1016/j.ogc.2014.02.005
0889-8545/14/$ – see front matter © 2014 Elsevier Inc. All rights reserved.

withdrawal and the high risk for relapse to illicit opioids.[3,4] When undertaken as part of a comprehensive care plan, opioid substitution therapy may result in improved access to prenatal care, reduced illicit drug use, reduced exposure to infections associated with intravenous drug use, improved maternal nutrition, and improved infant birth weight.[2]

Substitution therapy must aim for an appropriate buprenorphine or methadone dose regimen to encourage patient adherence to the treatment program.[2] In making dosage adjustments, clinicians should be guided by patient-reported craving and withdrawal symptoms.[2] The requirement for increased doses during pregnancy is expected because of physiologic maternal increases in weight, intravascular volume, and increase in renal elimination during the second and third trimesters.[2] The objective of this review is to describe differences in patient selection between the two drugs, their relative safety during pregnancy, and changes in daily doses as a guide for prescribing clinicians.

METHADONE
Dosing Regimen and Precautions

The authors have previously reported experience with 139 consecutively chosen patients requiring methadone; about one-fifth were already taking methadone before pregnancy, while dosing during pregnancy began at the following gestational weeks: 4 to 8 weeks, 25 (18%); 9 to 16 weeks, 46 (33%); 17 to 24 weeks, 36 (26%); and 25 weeks, 3 (2%).[2] Although it is the authors' practice to admit all patients to the antepartum hospital ward as early as possible for methadone initiation, other authorities believe that hospital admission is not necessary.[3,4] If patients are already receiving care in a methadone treatment program, pregnancy need not interrupt this therapy.[1] Methadone is available as an injectable solution or tablet, but is most often used as an oral solution.

Sonographic confirmation of a viable intrauterine pregnancy is often a prerequisite for acceptance to a methadone treatment program tailored specifically to pregnant women.[1] The initial evaluation includes a variety of tests. The authors suggest baseline tests for hepatitis B and C as well as liver function tests. Counseling regarding testing for human immunodeficiency virus (HIV) should be provided, and testing recommended using an opt-out approach. An electrocardiogram is recommended before beginning methadone because the drug can prolong the QT interval and cause torsades de pointes.[5]

The starting daily dose of methadone is as a single oral dose of 20 mg.[1] An additional 5 to 10 mg is given every 3 to 6 hours as needed for any signs or symptoms of withdrawal. Once withdrawal symptoms are suppressed, the dose should be increased no more frequently than every 3 to 5 days, to avoid overdose resulting from the long half-life of methadone (20–35 hours).[1] On the second day of treatment, the total dose of methadone given in the previous 24 hours is provided as the new morning dose. The patient's condition is considered to be stable when no remarkable symptoms or signs (dysphoria and restlessness, rhinorrhea and lacrimation, myalgias and arthralgias, nausea, vomiting, abdominal cramping, and diarrhea) are evident within 24 hours after her last dose. If the patient has been hospitalized for methadone initiation, she may receive the same single morning methadone dose as dispensed at the clinic pharmacy. Take-home doses are allowed over Sundays or holidays unless a random urine drug screen, performed at least monthly, is positive for other substances.

The authors' experience regarding daily maintenance dose ranges is similar to that of others.[2] The mean initial maintenance dose is 69 mg (range 8–160 mg) while the mean dose at delivery is 93 mg (range 12–185 mg). Nearly half require a low daily dose (<60 mg) while the remainder are maintained initially on a medium (60–89 mg) or high dose (≥90 mg).

As gestation advances, the dose of methadone usually increases rather than remaining the same (8%) or decreasing (6%).[2] This gradual daily dose increases during pregnancy (mean: 24 mg; 95% confidence level 20–28 mg) and is greatest when the initial daily dose is low. Doses are anticipated to remain essentially unchanged between 36 weeks and delivery.[2]

There is strong physiologic and pharmacokinetic evidence to support these observations about dosage requirements during pregnancy. Plasma levels of methadone decrease and renal clearance increases as gestation advances.[6] The half-life of methadone is reported to decrease from an average of 22 to 24 hours in nonpregnant women to as low as 8 hours in pregnant women.[6] These pharmacokinetic changes may result from prolonged gastrointestinal transit times resulting in increased absorption, decreased protein binding, expanded volume of distribution, and increased hepatic and renal clearance.[6] For those reasons, cravings often become apparent before each single daily dosing.

Split dosing of methadone during pregnancy has been suggested, although there have been no comparative randomized trials during pregnancy.[6] Twice-daily (or rarely 3 times daily) dosing is sometimes used in pregnant women and results in more sustained plasma levels, fewer withdrawal symptoms, and less illicit drug use.[7] Split dosing also does not suppress fetal neurobehavior (eg, body movement, breathing) as much as single dosing (see section on fetal and neonatal issues).[7,8] Twice-daily dosing is optimally delivered at 12-hour intervals, but is not possible for all women because it requires take-home doses.

There is a high degree of interindividual variability during pregnancy in methadone metabolism, signs and symptoms of opioid withdrawal, and desire by the mother to take more or less methadone. Some obstetricians wish to lower the methadone doses during pregnancy because of concerns about fetal exposure and severity of subsequent neonatal abstinence syndrome. Tapering methadone during pregnancy is not recommended, however, as it increases the probability of undesired maternal events. Such events include increased maternal opioid cravings and withdrawal symptoms, prompting patients to relapse on illicit drugs and potentially harm the fetus.[9]

The patient's usual oral methadone dose should be continued intrapartum. After delivery, fluid shifts may result in an increase of methadone levels. The authors continue the antepartum maintenance dose until discharge and have not experienced any cases of oversedation. By the sixth postpartum week, most patients (86%) remain within 10 mg of their dose at delivery (mean decrease in dose = −4 mg).[2] None were found to require a higher dose by 6 weeks postpartum than at delivery.

Ideally, during and after pregnancy patients should stay with supportive friends or family, and avoid contact with drug users and other triggers of relapse. Patients should be advised to avoid alcohol or sedating drugs. Any ongoing opioid use will delay the time to reach the optimal dose of methadone by building up tolerance. Those who insist on using drugs to relieve withdrawal symptoms should be advised to take the drug only when they are in severe withdrawal, at least 10 hours after taking methadone; use only the smallest amount of opioid necessary to relieve withdrawal symptoms, preferably by the oral route; and avoid alcohol, benzodiazepines, sedatives, antihistamines, and street methadone.

Effects on the Developing Fetus and Infant

Limited information exists about the risk for fetal structural anomalies with methadone exposure. One human study reported a small increase in congenital anomalies associated with methadone use, but numbers of individual kinds of malformations were small with no clear pattern.[10] Methadone did not produce teratogenic effects in pregnant rats and rabbits.[11] When given in large doses, methadone caused birth defects in guinea pigs, hamsters, and mice.[12–14] Exencephaly and central nervous system defects were the most common congenital abnormalities reported in those mammals.[13,14]

There are no studies on which to base recommendations for antepartum fetal surveillance of women on methadone maintenance therapy. In the authors' practice, women who consistently demonstrate good compliance by negative urine drug screens do not undergo routine antepartum fetal testing (nonstress test, biophysical profile score), unless there are additional indications for fetal surveillance (eg, preeclampsia, fetal growth restriction, preterm contractions). Studies in humans have reported alterations of fetal heart-rate patterns with methadone maintenance therapy.[15,16] Nonstress test patterns are less likely to be reactive when performed within a few hours after administration of a dose of methadone.[17–19] To reduce the risk of a falsely nonreactive nonstress test or nonreassuring biophysical profile, the authors suggest performing the test at least 4 to 6 hours after the woman takes her daily maintenance dose.[19] If daily testing is undertaken, the test should be done just before the methadone dose is given.

Maternal opioid withdrawal during pregnancy can temporarily affect fetal adrenal and sympathetic nervous systems and may be associated with stillbirth,[20,21] although an association between maternal detoxification during pregnancy and intrauterine fetal demise is not supported by a high level of evidence. Based on these theoretical considerations and observations that detoxification during pregnancy has been associated with a high relapse rate, detoxification has been discouraged during pregnancy.[4] There have been no published randomized controlled trials comparing opioid substitution maintenance with detoxification during pregnancy. A 2008 observational comparison of outcomes among groups of women treated with methadone maintenance or tapered methadone during pregnancy found better outcomes in women maintained on methadone.[9] By contrast, a more recent observational study found that newborns of mothers who were detoxified from methadone during pregnancy had a reduced incidence of neonatal abstinence syndrome (NAS) and shorter hospital stays in comparison with those whose mother's detoxification was not successful.[22]

Neonatal effects associated with chronic use of methadone include prematurity, low birth weight, microcephaly, jaundice, thrombocytosis, and arrhythmias.[10,23–29] As in adults on methadone, exposed newborns can manifest a prolonged electrocardiographic QTc interval.[30] There is growing concern about the effects of methadone on the developing eyes, including reduced visual acuity, nystagmus, delayed visual maturation, strabismus, refractive errors, and cerebral visual impairment.[29,31]

Perhaps the best understood methadone effect on the newborn is dependency with subsequent postnatal withdrawal. Symptoms commonly emerge by 48 hours after birth. The authors' reported experience confirms the lack of robust data suggesting that NAS can be predicted by the maternal maintenance doses of methadone.[2] A 2012 prospective cohort study did not find the incidence or duration of NAS to differ between infants exposed to doses lower and higher than 80 mg per day. A review of 174 births that included women using more than 100 mg per day did not find an association between dose and the incidence of NAS.[32,33]

Rates of breastfeeding are low among methadone-maintained women.[34] An estimate of the infant dose of methadone was a very low percentage of the maternal dose.[35] Reviewing this, the American Academy of Pediatrics and the World Health

Organization Working Group on Human Lactation classified methadone as being compatible with breastfeeding.[36,37] Some of the benefits include improved maternal-infant bonding and favorable effects on NAS.[38–40] It is questioned, however, whether reported quantities of methadone are sufficient to prevent or ameliorate withdrawal symptoms in addicted infants. Mothers can be warned to seek medical advice if exposed infants appear overly sedated.[37] NAS can occur after abrupt discontinuation of methadone, so women who wish to discontinue breastfeeding should be advised to gradually wean the infant from breast milk.[41]

Long-term effects from methadone on infant neurobehavioral development are complicated by other environmental and genetic factors. Infants exposed prenatally have shown high levels of behavioral disorganization using the NICU Network Neurobehavioral Scale.[42] Exposure to higher methadone dose levels is associated with the highest incidence of neurobehavioral findings.

BUPRENORPHINE
Patient Selection and Initial Evaluation

Buprenorphine has recently emerged as an alternative treatment for opioid maintenance during pregnancy. Buprenorphine functions as a partial agonist at the brain's opioid (μ) receptor, blocking the action of full opioid agonists at this site.[43] By contrast, methadone is a full agonist at the opioid receptor.[3] For the opioid abuser requiring opioid maintenance, buprenorphine has a better safety profile because of its ceiling effect as a partial μ agonist. Buprenorphine is less likely than methadone to result in maternal death attributable to overdose.[44] Buprenorphine therapy offers the potential advantage that it may be prescribed in the private office setting, and does not require visits daily or every other day to a federally licensed methadone clinic.[45]

Physicians who choose to provide buprenorphine maintenance treatment must first undergo training by completing an 8-hour approved buprenorphine Continuing Medical Education program, and must file a notice of intent to obtain licensure to prescribe buprenorphine.[3]

Patients undergoing consideration for buprenorphine maintenance therapy should undergo evaluation for hepatitis B, hepatitis C, HIV, and tuberculosis, in addition to the routine prenatal laboratory evaluations.[45] The Center for Substance Abuse Treatment recommends that before initiation of buprenorphine, patients have evaluation of baseline liver function tests because concerns arose in the past regarding buprenorphine-induced hepatotoxicity.[46] Recent reports of buprenorphine use in pregnant populations have not substantiated this concern. There is currently no consensus as to whether routine monitoring of liver enzymes is necessary. The authors recommend liver enzyme monitoring in patients with underlying hepatic disease.[47–49]

Clinical Trials of Buprenorphine Versus Methadone During Pregnancy

Several systematic reviews have summarized the body of evidence from observational and randomized controlled trials comparing the use of buprenorphine versus methadone during pregnancy.[50,51] In a recently published comprehensive review, Jones and colleagues[51] systematically reviewed the 3 existing randomized controlled trials comparing methadone with buprenorphine maintenance therapy during pregnancy. These studies included the Maternal Opioid Treatment: Human Experimental Research (MOTHER) study, a double-dummy, double-blind trial comparing methadone and buprenorphine among 131 pregnant women[52,53]; the Pregnancy and Reduction of Opiates: Medication Intervention Safety and Efficacy (PROMISE) study, the feasibility study for the MOTHER trial[54]; and a small single-site trial comparing methadone with buprenorphine.[55] In total, these trials included 185 pregnant women, 110 of whom received buprenorphine and 75, methadone.

In their comprehensive systematic review, Jones and colleagues[51] evaluated the following maternal outcomes: treatment retention, use of illicit substances during pregnancy, and illicit opioids present in drug screens at delivery. In the largest of the extant trials, mothers randomized to receive buprenorphine were significantly more likely to discontinue the treatment than mothers assigned to methadone (33% vs 18%, $P = .02$).[52] There were nonsignificant increases in participants assigned to buprenorphine who withdrew from treatment, compared with those assigned to receive methadone in the 2 smaller trials.[54,55] Of note, the subjects who did not adhere to the treatments were not analyzed on intent-to-treat principles in this trial.[52] The likelihood of positive drug screens during pregnancy was also compared.[51] The investigators noted that the percentage of women with drug screens positive for illicit opioids did not differ between the treatment groups in the largest extant study.[51,52] The smaller Fischer trial found that women randomized to buprenorphine were more likely than women randomized to methadone to have positive drug screens for illicit opioids during pregnancy.[55] None of the 3 randomized trials found any difference in the percentages of participants who used other illicit substances such as marijuana, cocaine, and benzodiazepines.[51] Although both the PROMISE and the MOTHER studies reported on positive maternal urine toxicology screens at delivery; neither showed any difference in this outcome between mothers receiving buprenorphine or methadone.[52,54]

Patient Selection, Dosing Regimens, and Precautions

Buprenorphine is available in single-substance preparations as well as in combination with naloxone. Combination products are so formulated to prevent diversion. During pregnancy, dosing with buprenorphine alone is recommended, although no adverse effects have been observed with use of the combination products.[45]

Many medical providers consider women with polysubstance abuse to not be candidates for buprenorphine; however, a safety advantage of buprenorphine in comparison with methadone is fewer dangerous drug interactions.[4] Some women with addictive diseases, particularly those using large doses of heroin or methadone, will find buprenorphine unsatisfactory for dampening their opioid cravings.[45] Active liver disease had previously been regarded as a contraindication to buprenorphine use. More recent studies do not support any adverse effects of buprenorphine on hepatic function.[47]

Buprenorphine administration to a patient who has recently used a full opioid receptor agonist may cause precipitated withdrawal symptoms if the buprenorphine dose is administered too soon and a full opioid-receptor (μ) agonist is still occupying the opioid receptor.[3] For this reason, it is recommended that the patient who is to be started on buprenorphine exhibit a Clinical Opioid Withdrawal (COW) score of 10 to 12 or greater (moderate withdrawal) before receiving her first dose of buprenorphine.[46,48,49,56] It is recommended that the first buprenorphine dose be administered 24 hours after last use of a short-acting opioid such as heroin or morphine, or 2 to 3 days after the last dose of a long-acting opioid such as methadone.[3]

Once the patient is in moderate withdrawal, the first 2-mg sublingual dose may be administered, with a second 2-mg sublingual dose available to be given within 1 to 2 hours as necessary to control the patient's withdrawal symptoms. After initial dosing, the patient may be given an additional two 2-mg doses to take home for use as needed during the initial 24-hour period.[3] On subsequent days, the buprenorphine dose should be rapidly titrated upward toward a target dose of 8 to 16 mg.[3,45] Buprenorphine is typically taken once or twice daily, according to the preference of the patient.[3] Because it is a partial μ-receptor agonist, buprenorphine has a ceiling effect at 24 to 32 mg, beyond which higher doses are not more effective.[45]

Buprenorphine induction carried out before fetal viability is appropriate for the office setting. After 23 to 24 weeks of gestation, the authors recommend a brief inpatient admission for initiation of buprenorphine. In the setting of a viable gestational age, continuous fetal monitoring while the mother is experiencing acute withdrawal symptoms is recommended.

As gestation advances, the physiologic blood volume expansion may result in a decreased effect of buprenorphine in advanced gestation; as a result, some women may require dose increases at that time.[51,52,54,55] For example, one published case series of 27 mothers who received buprenorphine during pregnancy reported that 70% of these women required a dose increase during pregnancy.[57] In this series, the mean dose increase over the course of the pregnancies was 5.9 mg.[57] By contrast, a secondary pharmacokinetic analysis of oral fluid, sweat, and plasma buprenorphine and its metabolites in 9 PROMISE study participants did not reveal any significant differences in tissue level between 28 to 29 and 34 weeks. However, levels of buprenorphine and its metabolites were significantly higher at 2 months postpartum than during pregnancy.[43]

Buprenorphine therapy, because of its property as a partial μ-receptor agonist, may pose challenges for pain control surrounding labor and delivery.[1,3,45] Because buprenorphine blocks full opioid agonists from the μ receptor, and because of its ceiling effects, pain experienced by women receiving buprenorphine may be more difficult to control. A variety of strategies has been proposed to overcome this difficulty. For labor, epidural or continuous spinal-epidural anesthesia is preferred. The patient's regular buprenorphine dose may be continued throughout with supplemental nonsteroidal anti-inflammatory drugs (NSAIDs) prescribed postpartum. For cesarean delivery, neuraxial anesthesia is preferred, as opioid-dependent patients may be at increased risk for airway compromise. A variety of modalities have been proposed for postoperative pain control, including spinal or epidural morphine, increased buprenorphine dosing up to 32 mg daily in divided doses, decreasing the buprenorphine daily dose to 8 mg and substituting oxycodone (1 mg buprenorphine = 15 mg oxycodone) or morphine (1 mg buprenorphine = 30 mg oral morphine) in divided doses, or using high doses of a full μ-receptor agonist to displace the buprenorphine from the receptor.[1,3,45] Respiratory monitoring should be carried out when high doses of full agonists are required. Most pain-control regimens will also incorporate scheduled acetaminophen and NSAIDs.

Effects on the Fetus

Buprenorphine is transferred to the developing fetus with observed umbilical cord blood to maternal blood ratios at delivery of approximately 0.4 to 0.5.[58] In animal studies, buprenorphine exposure has not been associated with any pattern of malformation.[59] The 2 randomized controlled trials that reported on this outcome reported no congenital anomalies in the buprenorphine-exposed neonates.[52,54] A recent systematic review of both the randomized and observational literature concerning prenatal buprenorphine exposure has reported no increase in congenital anomalies above the expected baseline.[53]

In a secondary analysis of the MOTHER study, Salisbury and colleagues[60] compared fetal heart rate tracings via nonstress tests before and after methadone versus buprenorphine dosing, and found that fetuses in the buprenorphine group had more fetal heart-rate accelerations and fewer nonreactive nonstress test results than fetuses in the methadone group.[60]

An analysis from a Norwegian clinical cohort of 139 women who received methadone (n = 90) or buprenorphine (n = 49) during pregnancy between 1996 and 2009 found that infants whose mothers were exposed to buprenorphine had increased birth weight, increased length, and increased head circumference when compared with infants of mothers exposed to methadone. After adjustment for covariates, the investigators found that only the increased head circumference remained significantly different between the groups.[61]

Behavioral assessment carried out in the neonatal period on infants born to mothers who participated in the PROMISE study showed no significant differences in neonatal neurobehavior measured longitudinally between postnatal days 3 and 14.[62] The much larger MOTHER study[63] evaluated neonatal neurobehavior among 39 infants born to women who participated in the trial, using the NICU Network Neurobehavioral Scale. The participating infants were assessed longitudinally between postnatal days 3 and 30. The infants of mothers who had been assigned to the buprenorphine group showed more favorable performance scores on several measures, including stress abstinence signs, excitability, overarousal, hypotonia, and self-regulation.[63] Whether these short-term findings will lead to improved long-term neurodevelopment is not known.

The 3 existing randomized controlled trials that compared buprenorphine with methadone evaluated several end points related to NAS, including the percentage of neonates born to exposed mothers who required treatment for NAS, total medication dose required for treatment, and time interval between birth and onset of NAS symptoms.[51] These 3 studies reported no significant difference in the percentage of neonates born to mothers receiving buprenorphine or methadone who required treatment for NAS.[52,54,55] Approximately half of the infants required treatment, regardless of whether their mothers received buprenorphine or methadone.[51]

Although the largest of the randomized trials, the MOTHER study, found no difference in the proportion of neonates who required treatment for NAS, they did observe that buprenorphine treatment significantly reduced the dose of morphine required for NAS in comparison with methadone.[52] In the available randomized studies, the duration of hospital stay for treatment of NAS and for all causes varied widely, likely owing to differences in neonatal management protocols.[51] However, the largest of these studies, the MOTHER study, found that buprenorphine, when compared with methadone therapy, resulted in statistically significant reductions in overall hospital duration and hospital stay for NAS treatment.[52]

Breastfeeding

The pharmacology of buprenorphine secretion into breast milk has been well studied. For example, one pharmacokinetic study found that the relative infant dose of buprenorphine and its metabolite norbuprenorphine in breast milk was less than 1% of the maternal weight-adjusted dose.[64] No adverse effects of sublingual buprenorphine on breast-fed infants have been reported in the literature to date. Current evidence suggests that the amount of buprenorphine in breast milk is insufficient to prevent NAS.[65] The Academy of Breastfeeding Medicine Clinical Protocol #21 endorses breast feeding in opioid-dependent women on maintenance with buprenorphine as long as there are no other contraindications.[66] Advantages and disadvantages of buprenorphine in comparison with methadone are summarized in **Table 1**.

Table 1
Advantages and disadvantages of methadone versus buprenorphine

Parameter	Methadone	Buprenorphine
Patient selection	Treatment of choice for patients with long-standing polysubstance abuse	Not as effective for patients with long-standing addition or multidrug use. May be ideal for prescription opioid abusers or new heroin users
Patient preference	Requires daily visit to federally licensed methadone clinic	May be prescribed in office setting with weekly or biweekly dispensing/prescribing
Treatment retention	Higher treatment retention in available randomized controlled trials	Higher rate of dropouts from treatment
Risk of overdose mortality	Higher	Lower (but not absent)
Risk of drug interaction	Higher risk of adverse event or death from drug interactions	Lower (but not absent) risk of adverse event or death from drug interaction
Starting dose	15–30 mg	2 mg
Target dose	90 mg	8–16 mg
Interval at which dose may be increased	3 d	Daily
Risk of NAS	Equal	Equal
Duration of NAS	Longer	Shorter
Breastfeeding considerations	Safe	Safe
Neurodevelopmental outcome in exposed children	Favorable	Less long-term information than with methadone; generally favorable

SUMMARY AND FUTURE DIRECTIONS

The prevalence of opioid use among pregnant women ranges from 1% to 2% to as much as 21% in select populations. Opioids cross the placenta easily, and dependent women experience an increase in obstetric complications such as low birth weight, preeclampsia, third-trimester bleeding, puerperal morbidity, meconium aspiration, and fetal intolerance to labor. Neonatal complications include narcotic withdrawal, postnatal growth deficiency, microcephaly, neurobehavioral problems, increased neonatal mortality, and a highly significant increase in sudden infant death syndrome. Although methadone has been the traditional treatment of choice for opioid addiction during pregnancy, buprenorphine may offer several advantages, including decreased duration of NAS and decreased hospital stay. By contrast, methadone substitution therapy may result in higher patient satisfaction and patient retention than buprenorphine. Buprenorphine may be the optimal choice for women with prescription drug abuse or intravenous drug habits of short duration, whereas methadone is the better option for women with long-standing multisubstance abuse histories and previous failed attempts at detoxification.

There is a need of more large randomized controlled trials comparing different maintenance treatments with longer follow-up periods for the mother and infant (ideally until 1 year). Other relevant conditions, such as nicotine exposure and concomitant use of other centrally acting medications and nonprescription drugs such as cocaine, alcohol, and marijuana, are important to control for in these investigations. Moreover, studies assessing the effectiveness of psychosocial treatments in conjunction with drug therapy versus pharmacologic treatment alone are advisable.

REFERENCES

1. Young JL, Martin PR. Treatment of opioid dependence in the setting of pregnancy. Psychiatr Clin North Am 2012;35(2):441–60.
2. Albright B, de la Torre L, Skipper B, et al. Changes in methadone maintenance therapy during and after pregnancy. J Subst Abuse Treat 2011;41(4):347–53.
3. Jones HE, Deppen K, Hudak ML, et al. Clinical care for opioid-using pregnant and postpartum women: the role of obstetric providers. Am J Obstet Gynecol 2014;210(4):302–10.
4. ACOG Committee on Health Care for Underserved Women, American Society of Addiction Medicine. ACOG Committee Opinion No. 524: opioid abuse, dependence, and addiction in pregnancy. Obstet Gynecol 2012;119(5): 1070–6.
5. Katz DF, Sun J, Khatri V, et al. QTc interval screening in an opioid treatment program. Am J Cardiol 2013;112(7):1013–8.
6. Shiu JR, Ensom MH. Dosing and monitoring of methadone in pregnancy: literature review. Can J Hosp Pharm 2012;65(5):380–6.
7. Jansson LM, Dipietro JA, Velez M, et al. Maternal methadone dosing schedule and fetal neurobehaviour. J Matern Fetal Neonatal Med 2009;22(1):29–35.
8. Wittmann BK, Segal S. A comparison of the effects of single- and split-dose methadone administration on the fetus: ultrasound evaluation. Int J Addict 1991;26(2):213–8.
9. Jones HE, O'Grady KE, Malfi D, et al. Methadone maintenance vs. methadone taper during pregnancy: maternal and neonatal outcomes. Am J Addict 2008; 17(5):372–86.
10. Arlettaz R, Kashiwagi M, Das-Kundu S, et al. Methadone maintenance program in pregnancy in a Swiss perinatal center (II): neonatal outcome and social resources. Acta Obstet Gynecol Scand 2005;84(2):145–50.
11. Markham JK, Emmerson JL, Owen NV. Teratogenicity studies of methadone HCl in rats and rabbits. Nature 1971;233(5318):342–3.
12. Geber W, Schramm L. Comparative teratogenicity of morphine, heroin, and methadone in the hamster. Pharmacologist 1969;11:248.
13. Geber WF, Schramm LC. Congenital malformations of the central nervous system produced by narcotic analgesics in the hamster. Am J Obstet Gynecol 1975;123(7):705–13.
14. Jurand A. Teratogenic activity of methadone hydrochloride in mouse and chick embryos. J Embryol Exp Morphol 1973;30(2):449–58.
15. Ramirez-Cacho WA, Flores S, Schrader RM, et al. Effect of chronic maternal methadone therapy on intrapartum fetal heart rate patterns. J Soc Gynecol Investig 2006;13(2):108–11.
16. Jansson LM, Dipietro J, Elko A. Fetal response to maternal methadone administration. Am J Obstet Gynecol 2005;193(3 Pt 1):611–7.
17. Archie CL, Lee MI, Sokol RJ, et al. The effects of methadone treatment on the reactivity of the nonstress test. Obstet Gynecol 1989;74(2):254–5.
18. Levine AB, Rebarber A. Methadone maintenance treatment and the nonstress test. J Perinatol 1995;15(3):229–31.

19. Anyaegbunam A, Tran T, Jadali D, et al. Assessment of fetal well-being in methadone-maintained pregnancies: abnormal nonstress tests. Gynecol Obstet Invest 1997;43(1):25–8.
20. Zuspan FP, Gumpel JA, Mejia-Zelaya A, et al. Fetal stress from methadone withdrawal. Am J Obstet Gynecol 1975;122(1):43–6.
21. Rementeria JL, Nunag NN. Narcotic withdrawal in pregnancy: stillbirth incidence with a case report. Am J Obstet Gynecol 1973;116(8):1152–6.
22. Stewart RD, Nelson DB, Adhikari EH, et al. The obstetrical and neonatal impact of maternal opioid detoxification in pregnancy. Obstet Gynecol 2013;209(3):267.e1–5.
23. Blinick G, Jerez E, Wallach RC. Methadone maintenance, pregnancy, and progeny. JAMA 1973;225(5):477–9.
24. Carin I, Glass L, Parekh A, et al. Neonatal methadone withdrawal. Effect of two treatment regimens. Am J Dis Child 1983;137(12):1166–9.
25. Kempley S. Methadone maintenance treatment. Pregnant women taking methadone should be warned about withdrawal symptoms in babies. BMJ 1995;310(6977):464.
26. Lim S, Prasad MR, Samuels P, et al. High-dose methadone in pregnant women and its effect on duration of neonatal abstinence syndrome. Am J Obstet Gynecol 2009;200(1):70.e1–5.
27. Hussain T, Ewer AK. Maternal methadone may cause arrhythmias in neonates. Acta Paediatr 2007;96(5):768–9.
28. Cleary BJ, Donnelly JM, Strawbridge JD, et al. Methadone and perinatal outcomes: a retrospective cohort study. Am J Obstet Gynecol 2011;204(2):139.e1–9.
29. McGlone L, Hamilton R, McCulloch DL, et al. Neonatal visual evoked potentials in infants born to mothers prescribed methadone. Pediatrics 2013;131(3):e857–63.
30. Parikh R, Hussain T, Holder G, et al. Maternal methadone therapy increases QTc interval in newborn infants. Arch Dis Child Fetal Neonatal Ed 2011;96(2):F141–3.
31. McGlone L, Hamilton R, McCulloch DL, et al. Visual outcome in infants born to drug-misusing mothers prescribed methadone in pregnancy. Br J Ophthalmol 2014;98(2):238–45.
32. Cleary BJ, Eogan M, O'Connell MP, et al. Methadone and perinatal outcomes: a prospective cohort study. Addiction 2012;107(8):1482–92.
33. Pizarro D, Habli M, Grier M, et al. Higher maternal doses of methadone does not increase neonatal abstinence syndrome. J Subst Abuse Treat 2011;40(3):295–8.
34. Jansson LM, Velez M, Harrow C. Methadone maintenance and lactation: a review of the literature and current management guidelines. J Hum Lact 2004;20(1):62–71.
35. Begg EJ, Malpas TJ, Hackett LP, et al. Distribution of R- and S-methadone into human milk during multiple, medium to high oral dosing. Br J Clin Pharmacol 2001;52(6):681–5.
36. American Academy of Pediatrics Committee on Drugs. Transfer of drugs and other chemicals into human milk. Pediatrics 2001;108(3):776–89.
37. The WHO Working Group, Bennet PN, editors. Philadelphia: Elsevier; 1988. p. 319–20.
38. Jansson LM, Choo R, Velez ML, et al. Methadone maintenance and breastfeeding in the neonatal period. Pediatrics 2008;121(1):106–14.
39. Ballard JL. Treatment of neonatal abstinence syndrome with breast milk containing methadone. J Perinat Neonatal Nurs 2002;15(4):76–85.

40. Abdel-Latif ME, Pinner J, Clews S, et al. Effects of breast milk on the severity and outcome of neonatal abstinence syndrome among infants of drug-dependent mothers. Pediatrics 2006;117(6):e1163–9.
41. Sachs HC, Committee On Drugs. The transfer of drugs and therapeutics into human breast milk: an update on selected topics. Pediatrics 2013;132(3): e796–809.
42. Woodward L, Wuick ZL, Spencer C, et al. Early neurobehavior development of the infant exposed to methadone during pregnancy. Pediatr Res 2006; 3571(2006 PAS Annual Meeting):318.
43. Concheiro M, Jones HE, Johnson RE, et al. Preliminary buprenorphine sublingual tablet pharmacokinetic data in plasma, oral fluid, and sweat during treatment of opioid-dependent pregnant women. Ther Drug Monit 2011;33(5):619–26.
44. Bell JR, Butler B, Lawrance A, et al. Comparing overdose mortality associated with methadone and buprenorphine treatment. Drug Alcohol Depend 2009; 104(1–2):73–7.
45. Alto WA, O'Connor AB. Management of women treated with buprenorphine during pregnancy. Obstet Gynecol 2011;205(4):302–8.
46. Center for Substance Abuse Treatment (U.S.). Clinical guidelines for the use of buprenorphine in the treatment of opioid addiction. Treatment Improvement Protocol (TIP) Series 40. DHHS Publication. No (SMA) 04–3939 2004.
47. McNicholas LF, Holbrook AM, O'Grady KE, et al. Effect of hepatitis C virus status on liver enzymes in opioid-dependent pregnant women maintained on opioid-agonist medication. Addiction 2012;107:91–7.
48. Komaromy M, Silver H, Bohan J, et al. New Mexico treatment guidelines for medical providers who treat opioid addiction using buprenorphine. Santa Fe (NM): New Mexico Behavioral Health Collaborative; 2012.
49. Kraus M, Alford D, Kotz M, et al. Statement of the American Society of Addiction Medicine Consensus Panel on the use of buprenorphine in office-based treatment of opioid addiction. J Addict Med 2011;5(4):254.
50. Minozzi S, Amato L, Bellisario C, et al. Maintenance agonist treatments for opiate-dependent pregnant women. Cochrane Database Syst Rev 2013;(12):CD006318.
51. Jones HE, Heil SH, Baewert A, et al. Buprenorphine treatment of opioid-dependent pregnant women: a comprehensive review. Addiction 2012;107: 5–27.
52. Jones HE, Kaltenbach K, Heil SH, et al. Neonatal abstinence syndrome after methadone or buprenorphine exposure. N Engl J Med 2010;363(24): 2320–31.
53. Jones HE, Fischer G, Heil SH, et al. Maternal Opioid Treatment: Human Experimental Research (MOTHER)—approach, issues and lessons learned. Addiction 2012;107(Suppl 1):28–35.
54. Jones HE, Johnson RE, Jasinski DR, et al. Buprenorphine versus methadone in the treatment of pregnant opioid-dependent patients: effects on the neonatal abstinence syndrome. Drug Alcohol Depend 2005;79(1):1–10.
55. Fischer G, Ortner R, Rohrmeister K, et al. Methadone versus buprenorphine in pregnant addicts: a double-blind, double-dummy comparison study. Addiction 2006;101(2):275–81.
56. Handford C, Kahan M, Srivastava A, et al. Buprenorphine/naloxone for opioid dependence: clinical practice guideline. Toronto: Centre for Addiction and Mental Health; 2011.
57. O'Connor A, Alto W, Musgrave K, et al. Observational study of buprenorphine treatment of opioid-dependent pregnant women in a family medicine

residency: reports on maternal and infant outcomes. J Am Board Fam Med 2011;24(2):194–201.

58. Bartu AE, Ilett KF, Hackett LP, et al. Buprenorphine exposure in infants of opioid-dependent mothers at birth. Aust N Z J Obstet Gynaecol 2012;52(4):342–7.

59. Reprotox. Buprenorphine. In: An information system on environmental hazards to human reproduction and development. 2013. Available at: http://reprotox.org/Members/AgentDetail.aspx?a=2726. Accessed January 27, 2014.

60. Salisbury AL, Coyle MG, O'Grady KE, et al. Fetal assessment before and after dosing with buprenorphine or methadone. Addiction 2012;107:36–44.

61. Welle-Strand GK, Skurtveit S, Jones HE, et al. Neonatal outcomes following in utero exposure to methadone or buprenorphine: a National Cohort Study of opioid-agonist treatment of Pregnant Women in Norway from 1996 to 2009. Drug Alcohol Depend 2013;127(1–3):200–6.

62. Jones HE, O'Grady KE, Johnson RE, et al. Infant neurobehavior following prenatal exposure to methadone or buprenorphine: results from the neonatal intensive care unit network neurobehavioral scale. Subst Use Misuse 2010;45(13):2244–57.

63. Coyle MG, Salisbury AL, Lester BM, et al. Neonatal neurobehavior effects following buprenorphine versus methadone exposure. Addiction 2012;107(Suppl 1):63–73.

64. Ilett KF, Hackett LP, Gower S, et al. Estimated dose exposure of the neonate to buprenorphine and its metabolite norbuprenorphine via breastmilk during maternal buprenorphine substitution treatment. Breastfeed Med 2012;7:269–74.

65. Toxnet. Buprenorphine. In: Toxicology Data Network, U.S. National Library of Medicine. Available at: http://toxnet.nlm.nih.gov/. Accessed January 27, 2014.

66. Jansson LM. ABM clinical protocol #21: guidelines for breastfeeding and the drug-dependent woman. Breastfeed Med 2009;4(4):225–8.

Smoking Cessation in Pregnancy

Sharon Phelan, MD, FACOG

KEYWORDS

- Smoking cessation • Pregnancy • Interventions • Strategies

KEY POINTS

- More than 400,000 deaths occur per year in the United States that are attributable to cigarette smoking, and the risks to the general public are widely known.
- The risk to women, especially those who are pregnant, is less commonly known.
- During pregnancy, smoking increases the risk of low birth weight infants, placental problems (previa and/or abruption), chronic hypertensive disorders, and fetal death.
- Cessation of smoking during pregnancy can decrease or eliminate the risk for these complications.

INTRODUCTION

More than 400,000 deaths occur per year in the United States that are attributable to cigarette smoking. The risks to the general public are widely known. The risk to women, especially those who are pregnant, is less commonly known. Smoking raises a woman's risk for cervical, breast, lung, and ovarian cancer as well as early menopause.[1] During pregnancy, smoking increases the risk of low birth weight infants, placental problems (previa and/or abruption), chronic hypertensive disorders, and fetal death.[2] It is proposed that much of this happens because of vasoconstriction with decreased uterine blood flow from nicotine, carbon monoxide toxicity, and increased cyanide production. Infants of smoking mothers have increased risks of sudden infant death syndrome, respiratory infections, necrotizing enterocolitis, otitis media, and asthma.[1] In addition, the female offspring of pregnant smokers are more likely to have a nicotine addiction in adulthood.[3] There are reports of smoking decreasing the incidence of preeclampsia. This effect seems to be a late-term effect of smoking and not caused by nicotine because women using noncombustible nicotine delivery systems do not have the same protection.[4]

The author has nothing to disclose.
Department of Obstetrics and Gynecology, MSC10 5580, 1 University of New Mexico, Albuquerque, NM 87131, USA
E-mail address: stphelan@salud.unm.edu

Obstet Gynecol Clin N Am 41 (2014) 255–266
http://dx.doi.org/10.1016/j.ogc.2014.02.007   **obgyn.theclinics.com**
0889-8545/14/$ – see front matter © 2014 Elsevier Inc. All rights reserved.

Risk factors for continued smoking during pregnancy include

- Less than 25 years of age
- Non-Hispanic whites
- High school education or less
- Unmarried
- Annual income less than $15,000
- Unintended pregnancy
- First-time mothers
- Late care initiation
- Enrolled in Medicaid and/or Women, Infants, and Children Program

MANAGEMENT GOALS

The intent of intervention is to cease smoking not only for the duration of the pregnancy but permanently. If this is not successful, decreasing the number of cigarettes used and exposure to secondhand smoke can provide some benefit for both a woman and her infant.[5]

The problem with intervention is that the most robust studies have been conducted in the nonpregnant population. Studies during pregnancy are small, often qualitative and descriptive, and difficult to generalize to the pregnant population.[6] Also, as is the case with many addictive behaviors, the motivation to smoke and to continue to smoke can be extremely varied from patient to patient. These motivations can include simple habit; social activity with family/friends; nicotine addiction; a weight loss tool; and self-treatment for depression, attention-deficit/hyperactivity disorder (ADHD), or other mental illness.[7] Attempting to address only the end result (smoking/nicotine use) versus the root cause for the behavior makes interventions variable in their success across populations. Most of the interventions for nonpregnant smokers have been suggested for pregnant patients, including advice; counseling; self-help material; nicotine replacement therapy (NRT); antidepressants, including bupropion; and pharmacologic cessation aids, such as varenicline.[8] Safety and effectiveness in this subpopulation of smokers is controversial. Most systematic reviews have reported limited effectiveness for most interventions during pregnancy or postpartum.[5] Overall it seems from systematic reviews done in Canada and the United States that NRT, incentives, self-help materials, and counseling do help with cessation success during pregnancy. The effects of these methods post partum are less clear.

In addition to the amount and duration of smoking by pregnant women (level of dependence), there are other predictors as to the likelihood of acceptance of intervention and success. Up to 10% to 40% of smokers will quit before their first prenatal visit.[9] Women who spontaneously quit before prenatal care tend to be less nicotine addicted, have more concerns about fetal effects, receive early prenatal care, have more nausea, and are more educated. These women are more likely to remain smoke free during the pregnancy.

Women who have smoked through prior pregnancies, have household members that smoke, use other substances or alcohol, and smoke in the workplace will have less success. Much like obesity findings, the influence of partners, family, and friends on success or failure needs to be acknowledged.[10] Women who are successful typically have fewer temptations at home and work, with more nonsmokers in the circle of support. The smokers who are seen as support people for these women are more active in their praise and staying smoke free when around them while pregnant.[11,12] However, this support may lapse once she delivers and no longer has the condition of pregnancy as a motivation. This lapse in support is probably part of the reason for the high rate of relapse within 6 months of delivery.

NONPHARMACEUTICAL STRATEGIES

The critical step to helping a pregnant smoker is to ask the question regarding smoking and nicotine use correctly. In the past, almost all women acquired their nicotine through smoking cigarettes. There seems to be a 25% nondisclosure rate during pregnancy. Now with the option of snuff, hookahs and e-cigarettes, the question has to be more open ended to include these "non-smoking" options. Since these alternatives are being advertised as a safe alternative to smoking, many women may not admit to using these noncombustible products. Without the clues of smoke odor on their clothing and nicotine stains on fingers, the provider may not otherwise become aware of this problem.

The foundation of the intervention in pregnancy is the National Cancer Institute's 5 As approach complemented with the 5 Rs (**Boxes 1** and **2**). This approach is scientifically based, doable in an office setting, inexpensive, and likely to have an immediate impact.[1,13,14] However, it is not time neutral and involves staff or outside resources (**Box 3**) to do the actual necessary counseling and education.

It should be noted that heavy smokers are not significantly helped by counseling only. They need to be offered medication intervention too. A multicomponent approach is more likely to be effective for the nonspontaneous quitter, but results are inconsistent. The SCRIPT trial (Smoking Cessation and Reduction In Pregnancy Treatment) demonstrated up to a 50% improvement in the cessation rate (nicotine confirmed) among pregnant smokers if multiple interventions including counseling, trouble shooting, and education occurred over the entire pregnancy rather than a single session.[15]

Box 1
National Cancer Institute's 5 As

1. ASK: standard multiple choice question to get a true picture of never smokers, recent quitters, those who have cut down since pregnancy, and those who have not changed behavior since pregnancy

2. ADVISE/educate: clear, patient-relevant message to quit and the benefits for her, the infant, and the rest of the family

3. ASSESS

   a. Past and current levels of smoking/nicotine use

   b. Willingness to stop within 30 days or resistance to quitting attempt (see **Box 2**)

4. ASSIST: through the stages of change, which can include education, counseling, and/or referral

5. ARRANGE: follow-up by asking at each visit how you can help

   a. If abstaining, praise

   b. If relapsed, identify the possible source and develop new approach and not see as a failure but learning opportunity

   c. If continued resistance, review the 5 Rs

Adapted from American College of Obstetricians and Gynecologists. Smoking cessation during pregnancy. Committee Opinion No. 471. Obstet Gynecol 2010;116:1241–4.

Box 2
National Cancer Institute's 5 Rs: for patients in the precontemplative or contemplative stage of change and unwilling to make a quit attempt

1. RELEVANCE to the patients' individual situation, finances, children at home, illnesses related to smoking/nicotine

2. RISK of smoking
   a. Ask patient what she knows about the risks of smoking, especially in pregnancy.
   b. Stress the benefits of cessation for her, her baby, and other family members.
   c. Just because other pregnancies were OK does not guarantee the same for this one.

3. REWARDS of quitting smoking for the individual situation
   a. More oxygen for baby (will get more oxygen within 1 day to help with development)
   b. More money
   c. Less secondhand and thirdhand smoke exposure for others
   d. Better-tasting food
   e. More energy

4. ROADBLOCKS or barriers to quitting
   a. Irritability
   b. Other smokers (family and friends smoking around her)
   c. Triggers (smoking with coffee after a meal) and cravings
   d. Weight gain
   e. Patient-identified barriers

5. REPEAT steps (at every visit)

Adapted from American College of Obstetricians and Gynecologists. Smoking cessation during pregnancy. Committee Opinion No. 471. Obstet Gynecol 2010;116:1241–4.

Over the last few years, a few studies have started to look at how to combine prenatal and postpartum smoking cessation programs to prevent the high rate of relapse during the postpartum period. There are currently no effective interventions known because of the lack of studies in this area. Should pediatric providers be involved? Would more frequent visits post partum similar to antepartum help maintain the support needed to be successful? These questions are important but unanswered.[16]

PHARMACOLOGIC STRATEGIES

In nonpregnant smokers, both NRT and antidepressants approximately double cessation rates compared with nonpharmaceutical methods (**Table 1**). There are no existing studies in which the safety or efficacy of either NRT or antidepressants has occurred with sufficient numbers of pregnant subjects to determine what might occur with large-scale use.[5] Studies have shown that only about 30% of obstetric providers discuss medication for cessation with smokers.[17] They then typically recommend NRT over bupropion 2 to 1. Only a third of patients follows through and uses the medication. Patients report fears of use during pregnancy, cost, or lack of confidence to succeed as their reasons for nonuse of these adjunct methods.[17]

Box 3
Web resources for smoke cessation training, information, and patient education (all verified January 8, 2014)

Resources for smokers and their families

1-800-QUIT-NOW http://www.smokefree.gov

Provides support in quitting, including free quit coaching, a free quit plan, free educational materials, and referrals to local resources for all smokers

Smokefree Women http://women.smokefree.gov

Provides information and resources targeted at pregnant and nonpregnant women

Smokefree.gov http://smokefree.gov

Provides general resources for smokers to quit

Become an EX: For pregnant and postpartum smokers http://www.becomeanex.org/pregnant-smokers.php

A program developed by the American Legacy Foundation

Stay Away from Tobacco http://www.cancer.org/Healthy/StayAwayfromTobaccoindex

Provides general resources from the American Cancer Society

Resources for providers

"Talk With Your doctor," Tips From Former Smokers http://www.cdc.gov/tobacco/campaign/tips/groups/health-care-providers.html

Campaign resources, including posters, videos, and factsheet

American College of Obstetricians and Gynecologists: Smoking Cessation http://www.acog.org/About ACOG/ACOG Departments/Tobacco Alcohol and Substance Abuse.aspx

Smoking cessation resources for patients and providers

Treating Tobacco Use and Dependence: 2008 Update http://www.ncbLnlm.nih.gov/books/NBK63952

Clinical Practice Guidelines, Treating Tobacco Use and Dependence. Is designed to assist clinicians; smoking cessation specialists; and health care administrators, insurers, and purchasers. This site also has clinician resources such as a Quick Reference Guide, tear sheets for primary and prenatal care providers, and consumer materials.

Smoke-Free Families http://smokefreefamilies.tobacco-cessation.org

Treatobacco.net http://www.treatobacco.net

Presents evidence-based information

"How Tobacco Smoke Causes Disease: What It Means to You" http://www.cdc.gov/tobacco/datastatistics/sgr/2010/consumerbooklet/index.htm

An easy-to-read booklet explaining new scientific findings

American Academy of Pediatrics http://www.aap.org/richmondcenter

Provides tools and resources to help clinicians to create a healthy environment for children, adolescents, and families

Training materials for providers

Smoking Cessation for Pregnancy and Beyond: A Virtual Clinic http://www.smokingcessationandpregnancy.org

An interactive Web-based program designed for health care professionals to hone their skills in assisting pregnant women to quit smoking; training available for free for a limited time (expires August 2014) (reproductivehealth/MaternalInfantHealth/PMSS.html)

The American Congress of Obstetricians and Gynecologists' Smoking Cessation During Pregnancy: A Clinician's Guide to Helping Pregnant Women Quit Smoking http://www.acog. org/About ACOG/ACOG Departments/Tobacco Alcohol and Substance Abuse/NEW

A self-study program describes evidence-based methods for screening and counseling pregnant and postpartum women who use tobacco

Centers for Disease Control and Prevention Tobacco Use and Pregnancy Resources http://www. cdc.govlreproductivehealth/TobaccoUsePregnancy/Resources.htm

NRT

Nicotine is the addictive active substance acquired by the smoker. Nicotine can be delivered through multiple vehicles (chewing gum, transdermal patch, and nasal spray) and at varying doses. These products are designed to provide nicotine replacement for nicotine cravings and then gradually be decreased over several weeks until the individual is nicotine free. This approach has been shown to clearly increase quit rates in nonpregnant smokers.[18] The success rate in pregnancy is not as great. It is unclear whether it is only being used on the heaviest smokers in which the success quit rate is lower, inadequate dosing is used, or it is not initiated by the pregnant woman because of fears of the effects of NRT on the infant or cost.[17]

Nicotine crosses the placenta throughout the pregnancy. In fact, the nicotine concentrations in the placenta, amniotic fluid, and fetal serum are higher than in the maternal serum consistently throughout the pregnancy.[19] It is clear that nicotine causes vasoconstriction and increased blood pressure. This alteration on blood flow on the maternal side of the placenta may also alter the placental fetal circulation through a direct toxic effect on the fetal cardiovascular system.[20] There have been associations noted between smoking and the occurrence of cleft lip/palate, but it is not clear that this is causative. Finally, newborns can experience withdrawal symptoms if exposed to heavy levels of nicotine during the pregnancy. Nicotine from any source has these risks. NRT should only be used as a means to stop smoking not solely as a long-term replacement therapy. Although nicotine is concentrated in human milk, breastfeeding transfers far less nicotine to the infant than smoking during the pregnancy. It is comparable with the amount of exposure with the use of snuff or secondhand/thirdhand smoke. Thirdhand smoke is the residue on clothes, furniture, and other objects that can be picked up by others when they touch the objects, such as an infant crawling on a carpet or held in the smoker's arms. One way to decrease this is to not use nicotine products within 1 hour of breastfeeding.

Bupropion

Bupropion is an antidepressant used for depression, attention deficit hyperactive disorder, and smoking cessation. There have been concerns raised about the possible association with congenital heart disease or persistent pulmonary hypertension with use in early or late pregnancy.[21] Repeated studies have not confirmed these associations. Other studies raise a concern of an association with the increased occurrence of ADHD. However, these studies did not control for ADHD in either parent or actual use of bupropion versus filling a prescription. It may be that women are self-medicating their ADHD with nicotine. This circumstance would create a greater risk of this in their offspring. With breastfeeding during use, there is no detectable drug or major metabolites in the infant's serum. The major concern with this medication is the risk of seizures, so it should not be used in patients with seizure disorders or

Table 1
Pharmaceutical methods for smoking cessation

	Dosage	Instructions	Warning	Side Effects
Nicotine gum or nicotine lozenges	1 piece q 1–2 h then taper 2 mg if <1 pk/d 4 mg if >1 pk/d Max 24 pieces/d	Use up to 12 wk and continue to decrease during time; use chew and park method	Do not eat or drink 15 min before use or during use	Mouth soreness and heartburn or hiccups
Nicotine patch	If >one-half pk/d start with 21 mg/d × 4 wk, then 14 mg/d for 2 wk, and then 7 mg/d for 2 wk If <one-half pk/d start with 14 mg/d for 4–6 wk and then 7 mg/d for 2 wk	Use new patch every morning Consider taking off at night, especially if bad dreams	Do not use if patients have severe eczema or psoriasis	Insomnia and local skin reactions
Bupropion, sustained release	150 mg every morning × 3 d and then increase to 150 mg/bid	Start 1–2 wk before quit date; use for 2–6 mo	Do not use in patients with seizures or eating disorders; do not use with monoamine oxidase inhibitors; note FDA black box warning of serious mental health events	Insomnia, dry mouth, vivid or abnormal dreams
Varenicline	0.5 mg every morning × 3 d, then 0.5 mg bid × 4 d, and then 1 mg bid	Start 1 wk before quit date; use for 3–6 mo	Use in caution in patients with renal disease, severe psychiatric diseases (FDA black box warning), and cardiovascular disease	Nausea, insomnia, vivid or abnormal dreams

Abbreviations: FDA, Food and Drug Administration; Max, maximum; pk, pack.

at risk of a seizure disorder. A black box warning from the Food and Drug Administration (FDA) was added recently regarding the risk of severe mental health side effects, including suicidal thoughts and behavior.[18]

Varenicline

This drug acts on brain nicotine receptors. There are no human studies done in pregnancy. For this reason and the number of side effects, this is not recommended for use during pregnancy. An FDA black box warning was added recently about the development of serious neuropsychiatric symptoms, such as hostility, agitation, depressed mood, and suicidal thoughts and behavior.[18]

Combined pharmaceutical therapy has been shown to be much more effective in nonpregnant patients. There are not adequate studies to support this approach in pregnancy given the risks of each of these medications.

SELF-MANAGED STRATEGIES

Given the high rates of nicotine use in the United States and the desire by many to stop smoking (one of the more common New Year resolutions), it is not surprising that there are several strategies for an individual to use. None of these have been confirmed to be effective in the nonpregnant population, much less during pregnancy.

Noncombustible Forms of Nicotine Delivery

E-cigarettes and snuff are recent additions to the fleet of nicotine delivery vehicles.[22] These methods raise their harm exposure risks/concerns. Smokeless products (snuff) from Sweden and North America have a less than 10% risk of traditional smoking forms of tobacco. It is felt that much of this may be the avoidance of the carbon monoxide and other chemicals and tars created by the combustion of the tobacco. Products made in other countries appear to have less production oversight. This increases the risk of contaminants in the tobacco or flavoring that may further increase the risk of use.

E-cigarettes are battery powered units that vaporize a liquid typically containing flavoring and nicotine. The unit typically consist of a mouth piece and two interlocking tubes. The far tube is the battery. The proximal tube contains the heating element which atomizes the solution and the reservoir of solution commonly called "juice". This consists of a solvent (propylene glycol and/or glycerin), flavoring and usually nicotine. When the individual inhales, the solution is vaporized into a mist.[23] Depending on the brand each cartridge is designed to produce up to 400 puffs which is equivalent to 1-2 packs of cigarettes. Although proponents of "vaping" state that the mist contains only steam, a study found potentially toxic and carcinogenic substances but at much lower levels than typical cigarette smoke.[24] Although these products are marketed as a safe way to help quit smoking, there are several significant concerns. These products may be entry drugs into the use of cigarettes and allow individuals to avoid the regulations that have helped to reduce smoking, such as age limits to purchase, FDA oversight, laws to prevent smoking in public places, and costs from taxations. The e-cigarettes are not federally regulated in any way at this time.[25] They can be sold in most states to anyone regardless of age. In fact, many of the flavors are designed to attract younger buyers. The use of e-cigarettes has double among adolescents between 2011-2012.[26] Because they are not taxed, the cost is much less than cigarettes. Finally, because there is no smoke but only "steam", they can be used in public places such as restaurants, work sites, and potentially on school campuses and in airplanes. These are legal strategies imposed on traditional tobacco products that have decreased smoking nationally.[27,28] Avoiding these barriers may allow the individual to not only continue nicotine use but also to perhaps increase their nicotine intake. Although like other nicotine products, such as gum and patches, the e-cigarette or snuff might help a person successfully quit all nicotine products, there are no studies that support this as a primary use.[29] E-cigarettes are not safer; they are less dangerous, which is a subtle but important difference.[30,31] They avoid the toxins associated with smoke, but it is not clear about the safety of the propellants, such as propylene glycol. This chemical is commonly used in food to retain moisture and in cosmetics. It is not marketed for products that are inhaled. In fact, for propylene glycol the product manufacturer's specifications specifically states it should not be used to create vapors or smoke because of concerns of respiratory irritation with inhalation of large amounts.[32] Nicotine poisoning is also a risk in young children who are attracted to the "juice" by its fruity smell. Given the lack of studies in the general population, it is not surprising that there are no data specific to pregnancy.[33] These products should be treated in the same way as other NRTs, which are listed as FDA category D.

Smartphone Applications

There are more than 250 applications for smoking cessation available for download. The issue is that there is no oversight regarding the accuracy of the applications and whether they follow recommendations based on the US Public Health Service's (USPHS) Clinical Practice Guidelines. In 2012, a study by Lorein Abroms looked at the most popular iPhone (47) and Android (51) applications to determine their approach to smoking cessation and their adherence to the guidelines from the USPHS.[34,35] Overall applications have a poor level of adherence to the guidelines, with only a few recommending calling quit lines or using approved medications. These applications are not specific to pregnancy but are directed to nonpregnant populations. There are no studies proving the effectiveness of these applications in nonpregnant patients, much less in pregnancy. There are studies that have shown a benefit for quit-smoking text messaging programs on mobile phones for the nonpregnant population.[36] These programs are very popular modalities based on the number of applications downloaded. More studies should look at how to optimize these popular uses of cell phones in the cessation of smoking in the pregnant population.

Exercise

In nonpregnant smokers, studies have shown that exercise can interrupt nicotine cravings. A Canadian study showed that 15 to 20 minutes of walking at a moderate pace is adequate to ward off cravings for nicotine. Exercising women reported less irritability, restlessness, and tension. This finding is encouraging as a possible intervention because it has several other positive effects. However, the study size was too small to make a definitive claim.[37]

EVALUATION, ADJUSTMENT, RECURRENCE

Before starting a smoking cessation/nicotine reduction program within a clinical practice, several steps should be taken[38]:

1. Identify resources within the community, such as hospital-based counseling, 1-800-QUITNOW help line, or cancer society.
2. Encourage office staff and other providers to engage with the program. Everyone in the office needs to be committed to helping a woman's cessation efforts. Having posters with information and resources helps stress the importance of cessation.

The office staff should have a consistent pattern of encouraging cessation at each visit, acknowledging accomplishments, and supporting those having difficulties.

3. Have appropriate educational material readily available in the waiting room and examination rooms. These materials should offer tips for success, benefits of cessation, and counseling/support resources.

4. Use the teachable opportunity. Because most smokers would like to quit, find reasons that resonate with them to quit (their baby is small, their other child has asthma, their parent has emphysema) and offer to help them with their efforts. Treat each relapse as an opportunity to learn and modify the approach to improve the chance of success.

There is an interactive program that can help providers and staff prepare for helping pregnant patients to quit. This program is a Centers for Disease Control and Prevention–sponsored Web-based program that is a virtual clinic. It provides interactive encounters with several different patients whereby the provider can try different statements and counseling styles followed by a reaction from the patients. There are also several resources, including short lectures on various aspects of smoking during pregnancy (see **Box 3**).[39]

SUMMARY/DISCUSSION

Recently, a comprehensive review of the literature and strategies proposed for cessation in pregnancy attempted to identify the most effective and feasible interventions.[5] Their conclusions included

- Combined multiple components have the best likelihood of success (90% probability).
- Selection of the components used should be based on the particular considerations of the clinical setting, patient characteristics, and resource allocation.
- Incentives work well but can be financially costly, and patients tend to relapse once the incentive is removed.
- Other successful interventions include personal follow-up, NRT, feedback about biologic measures, information, and quit guides.
- Harms data are rarely reported; but this should not result in a conclusion that interventions, especially pharmaceutical measures, or alternative delivery systems such as e-cigarettes are safe.
- All of the data are during pregnancy or immediately post partum, so long-term cessation outcomes or long-term outcomes for the infant are not known.

REFERENCES

1. ACOG Committee on Health Care for Underserved Women and Committee on Obstetric Practice. Smoking cessation during pregnancy. Committee Opinion #471. 2010.
2. Varner MW, Silver RM, Rowland Hogue CJ, et al. Association between stillbirth and illicit drug use and smoking during pregnancy. Obstet Gynecol 2014;123:113–25.
3. Stroud LR, Papandonatos GD, Shenassa E, et al. Prenatal glucocorticoids and maternal smoking during pregnancy independently program adult nicotine dependence in daughters: a 40-year prospective study. Biol Psychiatry 2013;75:47–55.
4. Wikstrom AK, Stephansson O, Cnattingius S. Tobacco use during pregnancy and preeclampsia risk: effects of cigarette smoking and snuff. Hypertension 2010;55(5):1254–9.

5. Likis FE, Andrews JC, Fonnesbeck CJ, et al. Smoking cessation interventions in pregnancy and postpartum care. Rockville (MD): Agency for Healthcare Research and Quality; 2014. Evidence report/technology assessment no.214. (Prepared by the vanderbilt evidence-based practice center under contract no. 290-2007-10065-I.) AHRQ Publication No. 14-E001-EF. Available at: www. effectivehealthcare.ahrq.gov/reports/final.cfm.

6. Seybold DJ, Broce M, Siegel E, et al. Smoking in pregnancy in west Virginia: does cessation/reduction improve perinatal outcomes? Matern Child Health J 2012;16: 133–8.

7. Holtrop JS, Meghea C, Raffo JE, et al. Smoking among pregnant women with medicaid insurance: are mental health factors related? Matern Child Health J 2010;14(6):971–7.

8. Fiore MC, Baker TB. Treating smokers in the health care setting. N Engl J Med 2011;365:1222–31.

9. Tong VT, England LJ, Dietz PM, et al. Smoking patterns and use of cessation interventions during pregnancy. Am J Prev Med 2008;35:327–33.

10. Christakis NA, Fowler JH. The spread of obesity in a large social network over 32 years. N Engl J Med 2007;357:370–9.

11. Koshy P, Mackenzie M, Tappin D, et al. Smoking cessation during pregnancy: the influence of partners, family and friends on quitters and non-quitters. Health Soc Care Community 2010;18(5):500–10.

12. Merzel C, English K, Moon-Howard J. Identifying women at-risk for smoking resumption after pregnancy. Matern Child Health J 2010;14:600–11.

13. Bowden JA, Oag DA, Smith KL, et al. An integrated brief intervention to address smoking in pregnancy. Acta Obstet Gynecol Scand 2010;89:496–504.

14. Albrecht S, Kelly-Thomas K, Osborne JW, et al. The success program for smoking cessation for pregnant women. J Obstet Gynecol Neonatal Nurs 2011;40:520–31.

15. Windsor R, Woodby L, Miller T, et al. Effectiveness of smoking cessation and reduction in pregnancy treatment (SCRIPT) methods in medicaid-supported prenatal care: trial III. Health Educ Behav 2011;38(4):412–22.

16. Gadomski A, Adams L, Tallman N, et al. Effectiveness of a combined prenatal and postpartum smoking cessation program. Matern Child Health J 2011;15: 188–97.

17. Rigotti NA, Park ER, Chang Y, et al. Smoking cessation medication use among pregnant and postpartum smokers. Obstet Gynecol 2008;111:348–55.

18. Cahill K, Stevens S, Lancaster T. Pharmacological treatments for smoking cessation. JAMA 2014;311:193–4.

19. Luck W, Nau H, Hansen R, et al. Extent of nicotine and cotinine transfer to the human fetus, placenta and amniotic fluid of smoking mothers. Dev Pharmacol Ther 1985;8:384–95.

20. Reprotox Data Base. Nicotine agent #1156. Available at: www.reprotox.org/Members/Printagentdetails.aspx?a=1156. Accessed January 2, 2014.

21. Reprotox Data Base. Bupropion agent #1238. Available at: www.reprotox.org/Members/Printagentdetails.aspx?a=1238. Accessed January 2, 2014.

22. Zhu SH, Camst A, Lee M, et al. The use and perception of electronic cigarettes and snus among the U/S/ Population. PLoS One 2013;8(10):e79332. http://dx.doi.org/10.1371/journal.pone.0079332.

23. Bertholon JF, Becquemin MH, Annesi-Maesano I, et al. Electronic cigarettes: a short review. Respiration 2013;86:433–8.

24. Medical Letter on Drugs and Therapeutics. Electronic cigarettes. JAMA 2014; 311:195.

25. Fairchild AL, Bayer R, Colgrove J. The renormalization of smoking? E-cigarettes and the tobacco "endgame". N Engl J Med 2013;1–3.
26. Centers for Disease Control and prevention. Notes from the field: electronic cigarette use among middle and high school students – US 2011-2012. MMWR Morb Mortal Wkly Rep 2013;62(35):729–30.
27. Benowitz NL, Goniewicz ML. The regulatory challenge of electronic cigarettes. JAMA 2013;310:685–6.
28. Center for Disease Contraol and Prevention. Trends in smoking before, during and after pregnancy – pregnancy risk assessment monitoring system, United States 40 sites, 2000-2010. MMWR Surveill Summ 2013;62(6):1–19.
29. Etter JF, Bullen C. A longitudinal study of electronic cigarette users. Addict Behav 2014;39:491–4.
30. Fiore MC, Schroeder SA, Baker TB. Smoke, the chief killer – strategies for targeting combustible tobacco use. N Engl J Med 2014;370:297–9.
31. Meier E, Tackett AP, Wagener TL. Effectiveness of electronic aids for smoking cessation. Curr Cardiovasc Risk Rep 2013;7:464–72.
32. Reprotox Data Base. Propylene glycol agent 1663. Available at: www.reprotox.org/Members/Printagentdetails.aspx?a=1663. Accessed January 2, 2014.
33. Palazzolo DL. Electronic cigarettes and vaping: a new challenge in clinical medicine and public health. A literature review. Front Public Health 2013;1:56.
34. Abroms LC, Westmaas JL, Bontemps-Jones J, et al. A content analysis of popular smartphone apps for smoking cessation. Am J Prev Med 2013;45(6):732–6.
35. Fiore MC, Jaen CR, Baker TB, et al. Treating tobacco use and dependence: clinical practice guideline 2008 update. Rockville (MD): Dept of Health and Human Services, U.S. Public Health Service; 2008. p. 165–73.
36. Whitaker R, McRobbie H, Bullen C, et al. Mobile phone based interventions for smoking cessation. Cochrane Datasbase Syst Rev 2012;(11). CDC006611.
37. Prapavessis H, De Jesus S, Harper T, et al. The effects of acute exercise on tobacco cravings and withdrawal symptoms in temporary abstinent pregnant smokers. Addict Behav 2014;39:703–8.
38. Developing an office-based smoking cessation program. Available at: http://www.acog.org/About_ACOG/ACOG_Districts/District_II/Developing_An_Office_Based_Smoking_Cessation_Program.
39. Tong VT, Dietz PM, England LJ. "Smoking cessation for pregnancy and beyond: a virtual clinic," an innovative web-based training for healthcare professionals. Journal of Women's Health 2012;21(10):1–4.

Substance Abuse Treatment Services for Pregnant Women
Psychosocial and Behavioral Approaches

Nancy A. Haug, PhD[a],*, Megan Duffy, BA[b], Mary E. McCaul, PhD[b]

KEYWORDS

- Pregnancy • Substance use disorders • Alcohol use disorder
- Smoking and tobacco • Psychosocial treatments
- Co-occurring psychiatric disorders

KEY POINTS

- In the United States, licit and illicit drug use during pregnancy is a significant public health problem, with potentially significant maternal and fetal morbidity.
- Universal screening for tobacco, alcohol and drug use should utilize empirically validated approaches to reduce identification bias.
- Comprehensive assessment of pregnant women who use substances is important to identify their diverse treatment needs.
- Psychosocial and behavioral treatments across a range of intensities and approaches have shown effectiveness for reducing substance use and improving fetal outcomes.
- Comprehensive service systems should address the high rates of co-occurring psychiatric symptoms, trauma, and other maternal and fetal health needs of this high-risk population.

Women who abuse tobacco, alcohol, and illicit substances during pregnancy are best served by comprehensive substance abuse treatment services to address their complex psychosocial needs and comorbid psychiatric conditions. Substance abuse treatment of pregnant women is more effective than legal action and highly preferred over criminalization and incarceration to optimize maternal physical and psychological health and to improve long-term outcomes.[1,2]

In the United States, licit and illicit drug use during pregnancy continues to be a significant public health concern. Based on combined data reported in 2011 and 2012 by

Disclosures: The authors have identified no professional or financial affiliations for themselves or their spouse/partner.

[a] The Gronowski Center, Palo Alto University, 5150 El Camino Real, C-22, Los Altos, CA 94022, USA; [b] Department of Psychiatry and Behavioral Sciences, Johns Hopkins University School of Medicine, 550 North Broadway, Baltimore, MD 21205, USA
* Corresponding author.
E-mail address: nhaug@paloaltou.edu

Obstet Gynecol Clin N Am 41 (2014) 267–296
http://dx.doi.org/10.1016/j.ogc.2014.03.001
0889-8545/14/$ – see front matter © 2014 Elsevier Inc. All rights reserved.

pregnant women between the ages of 15 and 44 years, an estimated 15.9% smoked cigarettes, 8.5% drank alcohol, and 5.9% used illicit drugs.[3] Among perinatal women, marijuana is the most frequently used illicit drug in the United States,[4,5] with medicinal cannabis representing a new and relatively unrecognized problem during pregnancy.[6] Abuse of prescription and nonprescription opioid analgesic medication during pregnancy as well as methamphetamine has also increased significantly over the past decade.[7–9] Substance use disorders (SUDs) among women of child-bearing age typically precede the onset of pregnancy and are highly associated with co-occurring mental health problems, such as depression and anxiety disorders, eating disorders, trauma, and posttraumatic stress disorder (PTSD) resulting from childhood sexual abuse and intimate partner violence.[10–12]

Perinatal substance use can have a substantial impact on the woman and her developing fetus. In a *Public Policy Statement on Women, Alcohol, Other Drugs and Pregnancy*, the American Society on Addiction Medicine (ASAM) outlined the potential harm from alcohol and other drugs during pregnancy: (1) teratogenesis; (2) obstetric complications; (3) intoxication risk; (4) behavioral effects; (5) drug culture involvement; and (6) withdrawal syndromes.[1] Because of the risk of adverse effects on fetal development, the drug exposure threshold for harm is lower during pregnancy. Prevention, education, and effective treatments for tobacco, alcohol, and substance use during pregnancy are essential.

In this article, nonpharmacologic components of substance abuse treatment services for pregnant women are reviewed, with a focus on salient psychosocial needs. First, screening and assessment procedures with demonstrated usefulness for women and specifically pregnant women are highlighted. Next, a range of psychosocial and behavioral treatment approaches of increasing service breadth and intensity is described. Empirically supported treatments that address the behavioral effects of SUDs during pregnancy are highlighted, such as difficulty with interpersonal, occupational, or social functioning; limited coping skills; poor self-care and inadequate nutrition; lack of early and regular prenatal care; family dysfunction and compromised parent-infant bonding. Treatment methods are also advocated that address mental health issues, including trauma history, and reduce exposure to dangerous situations associated with drug culture involvement, including criminal activity (eg, prostitution, theft, selling drugs); sexual, physical, and emotional abuse; violence; and sexually transmitted diseases.

OVERVIEW OF SCREENING AND ASSESSMENT PROCEDURES

ASAM policy recommendations state that high-quality, affordable, and culturally competent SUD treatment services should be made readily available to pregnant and parenting women and their families.[1] Pregnant women and their partners should be offered the highest priority for admission to available treatment slots. The treatment components of the ASAM recommendations include:

- Opioid agonist therapy for women dependent on illicit opioids
- Family-centered treatment, including education and treatment of domestic partners
- Evaluation and case management for substance-exposed children
- Childcare and transportation
- Adequate and appropriate facilities for the outpatient and continuing care phases of treatment
- Perinatal care that is nonjudgmental and sensitive to special needs
- Facilitation of maintaining the family unit and mother-child unit, with consideration of alternative arrangements as needed

- Child protection services as alternative placement when there is active SUD and absence of others able to fulfill the parental role
- Collaborative, interdisciplinary relationships and consultation among primary care, obstetric, family medicine, and midwife practices with addiction treatment providers
- Preservation of the physician-patient relationship in regards to confidentiality and reporting laws
- Screening, evaluation, treatment planning, and case management for co-occurring mental illness and personal history of prenatal alcohol exposure, fetal alcohol spectrum disorder, or fetal alcohol syndrome
- Reproductive and contraceptive counseling, including the effects of alcohol, nicotine, and other drugs on pregnancy and fetal health

In evaluating the level of care and intensity of service needed for placing patients with SUDs, ASAM offers revised patient placement criteria (PPC-2R), using a multidimensional assessment. The 6 assessment dimensions of this model and pregnancy-specific considerations are listed in **Table 1**. Placement decisions are guided by the presence and severity of issues within each dimension.

Pregnancy is a medical condition (ASAM dimension 2) that places the patient at greater risk for complications, necessitating a more intense level of treatment. Moreover, all of the other dimensions in the ASAM model may be exacerbated or complicated by pregnancy. For women with psychiatric illness or severe psychosocial problems (dimension 3), assessment should include the impact of these conditions on treatment engagement and whether or not specific mental health treatment is warranted. Pregnancy can aggravate or diminish the symptoms of co-occurring psychiatric disorders.[13] Psychological symptoms may result from hormonal changes, lactation, medications, or the stress of pregnancy.[14]

Key questions for assessment of substance-using pregnant women may include:

- Are the emotional, behavioral, and cognitive conditions part of the SUD or adaptive changes of pregnancy?
- Do the concerns seem to be separate problems with a previous history or recent onset triggered by substance use or pregnancy?
- Are the emotional, cognitive, and behavioral symptoms ameliorated or exacerbated by medical stabilization and pharmacotherapy?
- Are the symptoms in excess of what is expected, given the type and amount of substance used?

Mood instability, irritability, anxiety, depression, dysphoria, fatigue, and sleep disturbance may present during protracted withdrawal[13] but can also emerge during pregnancy. Thus, diagnosis of a mental disorder is complicated by pregnancy, intoxication, and withdrawal and may be easier to assess with a timeline once the patient is stabilized.[15,16] Although it is essential to diagnose and treat psychiatric illness, it is also important not to overpathologize pregnant women, who may already be experiencing distress and stigma related to pregnancy or their SUD.

SCREENING AND ASSESSMENT APPROACHES

Screening evaluates the possible presence of a particular problem, whereas assessment defines the nature of the problem, diagnosis, and specific treatment recommendations. Some pregnant women may underreport their substance use because of stigma and adverse consequences, and women from diverse ethnic groups may find the screening and assessment process intrusive or threatening. To improve

Table 1
ASAM patient placement criteria and pregnancy considerations

ASAM Dimension	Assessment	Treatment Focus
Dimension 1: acute intoxication and/or withdrawal potential	Assessment for maternal intoxication, management of perinatal withdrawal	Detoxification, pharmacotherapy, and preparation for transition to addiction treatment
Dimension 2: biomedical conditions/complications	Consider maternal health, obstetric complications, teratogenesis, fetal stress, and distress	Prenatal and obstetric care, medical stabilization. Treatment of maternal and/or infant physical health or coordination of services
Dimension 3: emotional, behavioral, or cognitive conditions/complications	Diagnose previous or current psychiatric conditions and screen for subclinical psychological, behavioral, or emotional problems that complicate treatment. Risk assessment for suicidality and psychosis	Treatment of co-occurring psychiatric disorders and coordination with mental health providers. Crisis management and safety planning
Dimension 4: readiness to change	Assess stage of change for reducing or stopping tobacco, alcohol, and illicit drug use. Determine motivation for change caused by external factors (ie, health of infant; avoidance of legal consequences), mandated treatment or coercion due to pregnancy, ambivalence for change, and presence of internal motivation	Motivational enhancement strategies to advance readiness and treatment engagement; psychoeducation and increasing problem awareness for patients in precontemplation and contemplation stages of change; behavioral techniques for patients in action and maintenance
Dimension 5: relapse, continued use, or continued problem potential	Assess potential for prenatal and postpartum relapse, coping skills, and psychosocial risk factors	Continued prenatal and postpartum care for mother, engagement of partner and family. Strengthen coping ability and parenting skills and provide relapse prevention interventions
Dimension 6: recovery/living environment	Determine social and family support and other barriers to engagement, such as substance-using partner or abusive environment	Case management services including housing, childcare, economic, employment, and legal assistance

Adapted from American Society of Addiction Medicine. Patent placement criteria for the treatment of substance-related disorders. Second Edition–Revised. 2001. Available at: http://www.ncdhhs.gov/dma/lme/UMASAM.pdf. Accessed February 27, 2014.

reporting accuracy and reduce patient discomfort, both procedures should incorporate instruments that have been adapted and tested on women in specific cultural and linguistic groups.[12] It is also important to reduce societal stigma and identification bias during screening and assessment. In northern California for example, Kaiser Permanente, the largest US managed care organization, implemented universal screening by administering prenatal substance use screening questionnaires and urine toxicologies to all pregnant women who enter prenatal care as a method for reducing identification bias.[17]

Self-administered and computer-administered instruments are found to elicit more accurate responses than face-to-face interviews with both the general population and specifically pregnant women.[12,18] Clinical practice guidelines for treating tobacco use in pregnant women recommend multiple-choice questions to improve disclosure.[19] For example, "Which of the following statements best describes your cigarette smoking? I smoke regularly now; about the same as before finding out I was pregnant; I smoke regularly now, but I've cut down since I found out I was pregnant; I smoke every once in a while; I have quit smoking since finding out I was pregnant; I wasn't smoking around the time I found out I was pregnant, and I don't currently smoke cigarettes."

Three brief screening instruments are recommended specifically for pregnant women: the TWEAK[20] and T-ACE[21] for at-risk drinking; and a modified version of the Perinatal Substance Abuse Screen (5Ps, **Table 2**).[22,23] Chasnoff and colleagues[24] adapted the 5Ps to include a smoking question, because women who smoke cigarettes in the month before pregnancy are more likely to use alcohol or drugs while pregnant. Similarly, women who continue to smoke during pregnancy have a higher likelihood of using illicit drugs, with marijuana being the most prevalent.[25] An assessment of associated risk factors (eg, depression, living alone or with young children, living with a person who uses alcohol or drugs) may also help to identify women who are using alcohol and drugs during pregnancy.[24]

A variety of empirically validated assessment measures are available; time constraints and staff expertise typically guide instrument selection. The Addiction Severity Index (ASI) and the Global Appraisal of Individual Needs (GAIN) can be used to assess change over time in alcohol and other drug outcomes, including psychiatric severity.[26] The ASI is a semistructured clinical interview widely used to measure psychosocial functioning in the context of addiction.[27] The GAIN is a biopsychosocial instrument, which can be administered either via pencil and paper or computer as a screener or assessment battery in various settings.[28] The GAIN measures the recency, breadth,

Table 2	
Screening for alcohol, tobacco, and substance use during pregnancy: 5Ps	
1. Peers	Do any of your friends have a problem with drug or alcohol use?
2. Partner	Does your partner have a problem with alcohol or drugs?
3. Past use	Before you knew you were pregnant, how often did you drink beer, wine, wine coolers or liquor? *Not at all, rarely, sometimes, or frequently?*
4. Present use	In the past month, how often did you drink beer, wine, wine coolers or liquor? *Not at all, rarely, sometimes, or frequently?*
5. Smoke	How many cigarettes did you smoke in the month prior to pregnancy?

Adapted from Watson E. Institute on Health and Recovery, Integrated Screening Tool. Cambridge (MA). Available at: http://www.mhqp.org/guidelines/perinatalPDF/IHRIntegratedScreeningTool.pdf. Accessed February 5, 2014.

and frequency of problems related to substance use (ie, severity, withdrawal, human immunodeficiency virus [HIV] risk, readiness for treatment, relapse potential, recovery environment, criminality, employment, and service use). An advantage of the GAIN is that it can be used for treatment placement guided by the ASAM PPC and for care planning. In obstetric settings, the self-report version of the PRIME-MD Patient Health Questionnaire[29] is a potentially useful assessment instrument for psychiatric disorders in pregnant women.[30] Results from this 3-page questionnaire can typically be reviewed by the treating physician in less than 3 minutes. The Mini-International Neuropsychiatric Interview (MINI) is a brief, structured interview for assessing *Diagnostic and Statistical Manual of Mental Disorders* (DSM) psychiatric disorders and SUDs[31,32] and is used in several studies of substance-abusing pregnant women.[33,34] The MINI is available in several languages and formats, including a 15-item screener. Thus, a variety of instruments and approaches are available for substance use screening and assessment, which have been shown to be sensitive and valid for use with pregnant women.

OVERVIEW OF PSYCHOSOCIAL TREATMENT APPROACHES

As described earlier, ASAM has developed PPC to help guide clinical decisions on treatment intensity, duration, and content. These PPC are, in turn, linked to 5 levels of care:

- Level 0.5: early intervention
- Level I: outpatient services
- Level II: intensive outpatient/partial hospitalization services
- Level III: residential/inpatient services
- Level IV: medically managed intensive inpatient services

The next sections review recent knowledge on treatment effectiveness and care recommendations at each level of care for pregnant women with SUDs.

EARLY AND BRIEF INTERVENTIONS (ASAM LEVEL 0.5)
Screening, Brief Intervention, and Referral to Treatment

Screening, brief intervention, and referral to treatment (SBIRT) is a comprehensive model for addressing alcohol and substance use in primary care.[35] SBIRT for pregnant women provides opportunities for prevention and early intervention with at-risk substance users before more severe consequences occur. The American College of Obstetricians and Gynecologists endorses SBIRT as a component of prenatal care delivery to pregnant women.[36] A recent report indicated that implementation of SBIRT is both cost-effective and significantly improves perinatal outcomes.[17]

Screening identifies the likelihood of substance use and helps to identify potential associated problems and the appropriate level of treatment. Brief interventions range from practitioner advice on the cessation of substance use to psychoeducational counseling and motivational interviewing techniques. Referral to treatment provides access to specialized services for pregnant patients, who require more intensive services, such as training in parenting skills.[36,37]

Smoking Cessation

There are several nonpharmacologic, psychosocial interventions for smoking during pregnancy: counseling, health education, feedback, incentive-based interventions, and social support.[38] A recent review and meta-analysis identified psychosocial interventions for smoking during pregnancy that significantly reduced the number of low birth weight and preterm infants. There are no adverse effects for mother or fetus from psychosocial interventions, and 3 studies[39–41] also reported an improvement in women's psychological symptoms (**Table 3** gives a summary). Another recent meta-analysis[42] suggested that tailored self-help materials (ie, written, video, audio, telephone, or computer-based) for pregnant smokers increase the odds of quitting over standard care.

Interventions Targeting Alcohol

For a comprehensive review of brief interventions targeting alcohol, see the article by Chang and colleagues in this issue. Stade and colleagues[50] reviewed psychological and educational interventions for reducing alcohol consumption during pregnancy. Only 4 studies met criteria as randomized controlled trials (RCT); little evidence was found to support intervention effectiveness. Gilinsky and colleagues[51] extended this review to include non-RCTs for alcohol-reduction interventions delivered to pregnant women during antenatal care. Similar to smoking cessation, the psychosocial interventions for alcohol included brief counseling, self-help manual, ultrasonographic feedback, and basic education. This review also showed minimal overall evidence of effectiveness for these psychosocial interventions, although there were positive finding in specific studies. O'Connor and Whaley[52] reported better birth outcomes among a group of nondependent alcohol drinkers who received a brief multi-session intervention during pregnancy compared with a control group. Effects of a brief single-session intervention for alcohol use during pregnancy were found if the participants chose abstinence as a goal and had participation of a supportive partner.[53] A 9-step cognitive-behavioral self-help manual given to women attending prenatal care, who had consumed alcohol in the past month during pregnancy, was associated with lower consumption and a higher alcohol quit rate compared with controls, who received information about the effects of alcohol use during pregnancy from clinic staff.[54] The intervention included social support, self-monitoring, and self-reward for quitting, in addition to stress management and relapse prevention techniques.

OUTPATIENT TREATMENT (ASAM LEVEL I)

Outpatient treatment is the most common treatment setting for women to receive services. ASAM level I typically consists of 1 or 2 weekly sessions of individual or group therapy.[12] Outpatient treatment can be used at various points across the continuum of care and is especially suitable for pregnant women with less severe substance use problems and greater resources, including housing, employment, partner, and social support. Whenever possible, providers who refer pregnant women to outpatient treatment should initiate contact with the agency to assist the patient in accessing services. Direct linkage (eg, scheduling an appointment with a specific treatment provider) can double the chances of the patient completing the referral, compared with advice alone and asking patients to make contact.[16,55]

It is especially important for practitioners to follow up on the outcome of the referral. Many patients are lost in the transition process, especially after detoxification at a different location and stabilization, because they may be feeling physical relief or psychological distress about their situation.[16] Pregnant and postpartum women who are younger, especially younger than 20 years, and self-referred (ie, without agency support) tend to drop out of treatment markedly sooner than women who are older and referred to treatment.[56] In addition, less social and psychological impairment

Table 3
Psychosocial interventions for smoking during pregnancy

Intervention	Description	Summary of Findings[38]
Counseling	Typically used to enhance motivation to quit, problem-solving, and coping skills Delivered in person by a range of providers, by telephone, interactive computer programs, or audiovisual equipment May represent a brief intervention (eg, <5 min) or more intensive treatment (ie, over multiple sessions)	More effective than usual care to support women in quitting smoking during pregnancy, particularly when combined with other strategies Unclear whether a particular type of counseling is more effective than others Increasing intervention intensity does not correspond to an increased effectiveness among pregnant tobacco users
Health education	Pregnant women are given information about the risks of smoking and advice to quit but not further support or advice on how to implement change	Health education alone does not seem to be sufficient for quitting smoking
Biomarker feedback	Feedback about fetal health status (eg, ultrasonography) or biological measurement of smoking to the mother	Assisted pregnant women with quitting smoking, especially when combined with counseling[43,44]
Incentive-based	Delivery of a financial incentive (eg, gift certificate or voucher) to women contingent on reductions or cessation of smoking behavior	Had the most evidence for supporting women in quitting smoking during pregnancy, especially when provided intensively[45–48]
Social support	Involves support from a peer or partner to promote smoking cessation	Evidence for social support interventions was mixed in the smoking review, but they seem effective when provided by peers A qualitative review suggests that partners are an important influence on women's smoking and relapse, and can serve as both facilitators and barriers to quitting[49]

is associated with not entering treatment among pregnant and postpartum cocaine-abusing women.[57] Fewer psychosocial problems may be associated with minimizing the impact of drug use and lower motivation.

Strengthening motivation for change is promoted by therapeutic acceptance, hope, and compassion, not rejection or judgment. Miller and Rollnick recommend helping clients to recognize their own goals and values, by highlighting the discrepancy between their values and current reality, and how substance use impedes achievement of goals.[58] Other important aspects of treatment access are convenience of the outpatient program, including transportation and wait time.

Several psychosocial and behavioral treatment approaches have been shown to be effective when delivered in an outpatient substance abuse treatment setting (**Table 4**, ASAM level 1 outpatient psychosocial and behavioral treatments). Efficacy and effectiveness studies specific to women, and particularly pregnant women, are more limited.

Motivational Interviewing

Findings from motivational interviewing (MI) research with pregnant women have been equivocal. In 1 small-scale study,[76] a 1-hour MI session involving empathetic, client-centered feedback was associated with a reduction in alcohol drinking by pregnant women who had the highest blood alcohol concentrations during early pregnancy compared with women who received informational letters only. In contrast, a 30-minute MI session with components of establishing empathy, developing discrepancy, rolling with resistance, and supporting self-efficacy was not effective in decreasing prenatal drinking.[77] Moreover, MI interventions have not been associated with behavior change in low-income pregnant women who smoke[39,78–82] or abuse illicit drugs.[83,84] Another recent study[34] concluded that motivational enhancement therapy (MET) plus cognitive-behavioral therapy (CBT) had similar results to brief advice alone in reducing use of illicit drugs and alcohol among perinatal women recruited from prenatal sites. These investigators suggested that brief advice is efficient and can be easily integrated with prenatal care, whereas MET and CBT may be more suited for chronic and severe substance abuse.

Contingency Management

In general, contingency management (CM) approaches (also known as motivational incentives) have shown effectiveness for improving retention and drug abstinence among substance abusers in treatment,[82] thereby allowing patients to benefit from other components of clinical services. CM is of particular relevance during a time-limited window of opportunity such as pregnancy, in which longer treatment duration results in better maternal and infant outcomes.[85–87] CM interventions have consistently been shown to improve retention in drug abuse treatment and access to prenatal services for pregnant women, However, despite early promising support for the usefulness of CM to reduce illicit substance use in pregnant women,[88–90] more current reports have generally not found effects on substance use outcomes.[84,91] Nonetheless, a recent randomized clinical trial of CM versus a noncontingent voucher control did find higher rates of cocaine-negative urine tests and longer duration of cocaine abstinence among pregnant and postpartum women who received CM treatment.[60] The cost of CM programs makes clinical application challenging in community-based treatment clinics. Moreover, stigma and related negative public perceptions of paying women to abstain from substance use during pregnancy are often difficult to overcome.[85]

Table 4
ASAM level I outpatient psychosocial and behavioral treatments

Treatment	Description	Typical Number of Sessions	Manual or Protocol	Evidence for Application with Pregnant Women
TSF and mutual help groups (eg, AA, NA)	TSF is a manualized, structured approach based on the 12 steps of AA with emphasis on steps 1–5 Predicated on the theory of alcoholism as a spiritual and medical disease Goals are abstinence from alcohol and commitment to participation in AA	12–15	Nowinski J, Baker S. The twelve step facilitation handbook: a systematic approach to recovery from substance dependence[59] Self-help or mutual help groups include AA, NA, Self-Management and Recovery Training, Secular Organizations for Sobriety (SOS), and Moderation Management (MM) Women for Sobriety, a self-help approach for women, may be indicated for pregnant women. This group emphasizes women-specific issues, such as assertiveness, self-confidence, and autonomy	TSF does not seem to be superior to other evidence-based outpatient treatment approaches in pregnant cocaine-dependent women[60] Among persons with alcohol use disorders who contacted an information and referral service, women were more likely to attend AA and achieve remission than men. Women also showed greater reductions in depression and avoidance coping from extended participation in AA, compared with men[61]
CBT	Based on principles of social learning theory, alcohol and drug use are treated as maladaptive coping strategies Addresses a broad spectrum of problems (eg, interpersonal, intrapersonal anger, depression) Focuses on skill deficits and increasing coping ability in high-risk situations Related approach integrates cognitive-behavioral, motivational interviewing, and relapse prevention techniques in a group context[63]	12	Kadden R, Carroll K, Donovan D, et al. Cognitive-behavioral coping skills therapy manual: a clinical research guide for therapists treating individuals with alcohol abuse and dependence[62] Sobell LC, Sobell MB. Group therapy for substance use disorders: a motivational cognitive-behavioral approach[63]	Not tested in pregnant substance-abusing women, but CBT is widely used among other female populations, including pregnant women with depression[64,65]

MI/MET	4	Based on principles of motivational psychology and designed to produce rapid, internally motivated change Uses nonconfrontational strategies to mobilize the client's own resources MET is an adaptation of MI, and includes 4 individualized treatment sessions involving normative assessment feedback, resolving ambivalence, and promoting self-efficacy	Miller WR, Zweben A, Diclemente C, et al. Motivational enhancement therapy: a clinical research guide for therapists treating individuals with alcohol abuse and dependence[66] Miller WR. Motivational enhancement therapy with drug abusers[67] Applications of motivational interviewing are described in detail in Miller WR & Rollnick S. Motivational Interviewing: Helping People Change (3rd Ed.)[58]	Equivocal effectiveness for decreasing alcohol and substance use in pregnant women
Contingency management	8–12 wk (but can be modified)	Based on principles of operant conditioning in which behavior is modified by consequences Uses reinforcement to modify substance use Awards prizes, cash, or vouchers for drug abstinence, program attendance, and health behaviors Can be used as an adjunct to other forms of treatment in community-based settings	Petry NM, Stitzer M. Contingency management: using motivational incentives to improve drug abuse treatment[68] Petry NM. Contingency management for substance abuse treatment: a guide to implementing this evidence-based practice[69]	Has been applied successfully with pregnant women to increase retention in substance abuse treatment
BCT	15–20	Designed for married or cohabitating couples seeking treatment of substance abuse Goals are to decrease substance use, build support for abstinence, and improve relationship functioning Includes a recovery contract between partners and therapist	O'Farrell T, Fals-Stewart T. Behavioral couples therapy for alcoholism and drug abuse[70] Fals-Stewart T, O'Farrell T, Birchler G, et al. Behavioral couples therapy for drug abuse and alcoholism: a 12 step manual (2nd edition)[71]	In women, BCT decreases alcohol and drug use and increases marital happiness compared with IT.[72,73] Women with worse relationship functioning at baseline improved more in BCT compared with IT[74] Rates of intimate partner violence also declined for women in BCT; the decline persisted for ≥2 y[75] Not tested in pregnant substance-abusing women

Abbreviations: AA, Alcoholics Anonymous; BCT, behavioral couples therapy; CBT, cognitive-behavioral therapy; IT, individual therapy; MET, motivational enhancement therapy; MI, motivational interviewing; NA, Narcotics Anonymous; TSF, 12-step facilitation.

CASE MANAGEMENT AND OTHER SUPPORTIVE SERVICES

Pregnant women may require additional case management services or referral to other community supportive services to address their diverse needs as part of comprehensive outpatient treatment. Case management facilitates attendance in outpatient treatment, which in turn improves maternal and infant outcomes.[92]

Integrated clinical and community services should incorporate medical services, health promotion, psychoeducation, gender-specific needs, culture and language needs, life skills, family-related and child-related services, comprehensive case management, mental health services, disability services, and staff and program development (**Table 5**).[12] Ashley and colleagues[11] define substance abuse treatment programming for women as the delivery of services that: (1) reduce women's barriers to entering substance abuse treatment and (2) address the treatment needs specific to women. These investigators emphasize how services are delivered, in addition to the specific type or quantity of services. Specifically, this consists of a nurturing and supportive group therapy environment, focus on self-worth, and a comfortable setting for women to discuss sensitive and painful issues. An empirical literature review also indicated improved service use and outcomes when substance abuse treatment and child welfare services are integrated.[93]

INTENSIVE OUTPATIENT TREATMENT/PARTIAL HOSPITALIZATION (ASAM LEVEL II)

Intensive outpatient treatment (IOP) offers a higher level of care than traditional outpatient programs, without a structured residential living environment. IOP provides multidimensional services with step-up and step-down levels of care that vary in intensity and duration. Pregnant women in IOP typically receive between 9 and 30 contact hours per week with the following services adapted to their needs:

- Comprehensive biopsychosocial assessment
- Group, individual, and family counseling
- Psychoeducational programming
- Pharmacotherapy and medication management
- Ambulatory detoxification
- 24-hour crisis coverage
- Integration into support groups
- Relapse prevention training
- Substance use screening and monitoring
- Case management
- Vocational and educational services
- Childcare and parenting training
- Outreach and transportation

IOP treatment approaches integrate multiple evidence-based treatment interventions, such as the ones listed in **Table 4**.[94,95] In 1 early report, rates of treatment completion were higher for postpartum cocaine-abusing women in IOP compared with women in traditional outpatient treatment (45% vs 21%, respectively).[96] Recent research has examined strategies to improve retention and treatment outcomes for pregnant women in IOP care. For example, reinforcement-based treatment (RBT), modeled on the community reinforcement approach, provides abstinence-contingent access to housing, recreational activities, and skills training for employment in combination with typical IOP care. RBT significantly increased length of stay in substance abuse treatment and recovery housing for pregnant women with

Table 5
Substance abuse treatment service needs for women

Medical services	Gynecologic care Family planning Prenatal care Pediatric care HIV/AIDS services Treatment of infectious diseases Smoking cessation treatment
Health promotion	Nutritional counseling Education on reproductive health Wellness programs Education on sleep and dental hygiene Education about sexually transmitted diseases and other infectious diseases Preventive health care education
Psychoeducation	Sexuality education Assertiveness skills training Effects of alcohol and drugs on prenatal and child development Prenatal education
Gender-specific needs	Women-only programming Lesbian services
Cultural and language needs	Culturally appropriate programming Availability of interpreter services or treatment services in native language
Life skills	Money management and budgeting Stress reduction and coping skills training
Family-related and child-related services	Childcare services, including homework assistance in conjunction with outpatient services Children's programming, including nurseries and preschool programs Family treatment services including psychoeducation surrounding addiction and its impact on family functioning Couples counseling and relationship enrichment recovery groups Parent/child services, including developmentally age-appropriate programs for children and education for mothers about child safety; parenting education; nutrition; children's substance abuse prevention curriculum; and children's mental health needs, including recreational activities, school, and other related activities
Comprehensive case management	Linkages to welfare system, employment opportunities, and housing Integration of stipulations from child welfare, temporary assistance for needy families, probation and parole, and other systems Intensive case management, including case management for children Transportation services Domestic violence services, including referral to safe houses Legal services Assistance in establishing financial arrangements or accessing funding for treatment services Assistance in obtaining General Education Development or further education, career counseling, and vocational training, including job readiness training to prepare women to leave the program and support themselves and their families Assistance in locating appropriate housing in preparation for discharge, including referral to transitional living or supervised housing

(*continued on next page*)

Table 5 (continued)	
Mental health services	Trauma-informed and trauma-specific services Eating disorder and nutrition services Treatment of co-occurring disorders Children's mental health services
Disability services	Strong female role models Peer support Adequate staffing to meet added program demands Gender-specific programming Cultural competence concerning parenting style, discipline, children's diet, parental supervision, and adherence to medical treatment Flexible scheduling and staff coordination Adequate time for parent-child bonding and interactions Administrative commitment to addressing the unique needs of pregnant women in treatment Staff training and administrative policies to support integration with opioid pharmacotherapy Culturally appropriate programming that matches socialization and cultural practices for women

From Center for Substance Abuse Treatment. Substance abuse treatment: addressing the specific needs of women. Treatment improvement protocol (TIP) series 51. DHHS Publication No. (SMA) 09-4426. Rockville (MD): Substance Abuse and Mental Health Services Administration; 2009; with permission.

opioid or cocaine use disorders and reduced length of postdelivery hospitalization for their neonates.[97]

RESIDENTIAL AND INPATIENT TREATMENT (ASAM LEVEL III)

Through federal law, pregnant women are granted priority admission into residential treatment and immediate access when a bed is available. Comprehensive care for pregnant women includes substance abuse treatment, obstetric care, and pediatric care for the duration of pregnancy and postpartum. As is true at less intensive levels of care, longer stays in treatment of pregnant and postpartum women are associated with better outcomes.[98,99] Residential and inpatient treatment offers a safe environment for stabilization, structure, and intense support for recovery, in addition to the services listed in **Table 4**.[12] The Therapeutic Community is a residential treatment model which has been adapted to serve the needs of women (**Table 6**).[100] Pregnant women who live in drug-using environments may especially benefit from residential versus outpatient treatment.[101] In addition, lower infant morbidity and mortality have been reported among pregnant substance-abusing women in comprehensive residential treatment compared with untreated comparison groups.[102,103]

Collaboration among providers and having onsite nursing resources are important components of residential treatment of pregnant women. Women with a history of sexual trauma should preferably have a female obstetrician or female prenatal care provider as well as a labor coach or supportive individual to accompany them on medical visits and during labor and delivery.[12] When involving a partner in treatment of pregnant substance-abusing women, clinicians should consider the woman's safety and the partner's willingness to participate, along with history of violence, substance use in the relationship, partner's history of substance use, accessibility, mental illness, relationship support, and commitment to the relationship.[12,109]

Table 6
ASAM level III residential and inpatient psychosocial and behavioral treatments

Treatment	Description	Typical Duration	Manual or Protocol	Evidence for Application with Pregnant Women
TC	Abstinence-based residential treatment that uses a hierarchical model, with stages that reflect increased levels of personal and social responsibility Peer influence and group process is used to assist individuals learn and assimilate social norms and develop more effective social skills Referred to as community as method, because TC members interact to influence attitudes, perceptions, and behaviors associated with substance use Model adapted for pregnant and postpartum women in residential treatment	90 d (minimum); 18–24 mo preferred	Center for Substance Abuse Treatment. Therapeutic Community Curriculum: Participant's Manual[104] De Leon G. The therapeutic community: theory, model, and method[105]	When randomly assigned, women refused treatment admission and had higher dropout rates for TC services compared with short-term outpatient services regardless of whether services were cogender or women only[106]
Modified therapeutic community for persons with co-occurring disorders	Developed for individuals with co-occurring SUDs and mental disorders Adapts TC in response to psychiatric symptoms, cognitive impairment, and level of functioning Flexible, less intense, and more personalized than TC model	12–18 mo	Sacks S, De Leon G, Bernhardt A, et al. Modified therapeutic community for homeless mentally ill chemical abusers: treatment manual[107] Sacks SS, Sacks JY, De Leon G. Treatment for MICAs: design and implementation of the modified TC[108]	Not tested in pregnant women

Abbreviation: TC, therapeutic community.

Women-only treatment services are associated with increased length of stay compared with mixed-gender substance abuse treatment programs.[11,110] In addition, treatment focused on gender-specific needs results in longer stays and improved continuity of care.[111,112] Specialized services in residential treatment of pregnant women encompass:

- Nutrition services
- Prenatal care
- Transportation to obstetric appointments
- Childbirth education and preparation and a coach, if possible
- Mental health evaluation at least twice during the pregnancy and postpartum periods, and treatment as needed to rule out (or treat) postpartum depression or other disorders
- Education about alcohol and drug use specifically related to pregnancy, including education about neonatal abstinence syndrome and, if possible, a tour of the nursery in the delivery site for the woman in anticipation of the need for infant monitoring in the hospital
- Education about HIV/AIDS risk and management during pregnancy, especially because HIV/AIDS transmission to the fetus and infants can be prevented
- Education about breastfeeding and strong support for mothers who nurse their babies, unless they are HIV positive

Research suggests that women become more engaged, obtain greater benefit from treatment, and have higher retention when they are permitted to bring their children into the residential treatment setting.[113–117] Women in residential treatment with their children have better outcomes across multiple areas of psychosocial functioning at 6 months after discharge (ie, drug abstinence, employment, child custody, and involvement with continuing care and support groups) than women who do not bring their children to treatment.[118] Moreover, improved behavioral and emotional functioning at 6 and 12 months after residential treatment was found among children who attended residential treatment with their mothers.[119]

ANCILLARY TREATMENTS FOR PREGNANT WOMEN WITH SUDS
Psychiatric Treatment

Multiple studies have shown high rates of psychiatric comorbidity (64%–75% DSM-IV axis I disorders) among pregnant women who are dependent on alcohol, opioids, or stimulants.[9,120–123] The severity and complexity of co-occurring mental disorders influence the level and intensity of substance abuse treatment of pregnant women.[13] Previous psychiatric hospitalization and severe psychopathology are associated with poor retention in treatment by pregnant cocaine-abusing women.[124,125] Similarly, pregnant opioid-dependent women with anxiety or depressive symptoms are at higher risk for discontinuing treatment than women without symptoms.[33,122] Tuten and colleagues[126] reported that pregnant opioid-dependent women with co-occurring psychiatric disorders also were more likely to test positive for illicit substances during treatment. Furthermore, infants born to methadone-maintained mothers with mood disorders had longer neonatal intensive care unit stays than those whose mothers did not show comorbid mood symptoms. Depressive symptoms and major depressive disorder are independent predictors of continued smoking during pregnancy.[127] Smoking behavior in pregnancy may also be influenced by abuse-related PTSD symptoms.[128] Clearly, pregnant women with co-occurring disorders require psychiatric services in conjunction with substance abuse treatment to improve maternal and infant outcomes. One residential treatment program,[98] which included mental health services, reduced symptoms of depression and PTSD in primarily methamphetamine-abusing and cocaine-abusing pregnant women.

Trauma Services

Women with SUDs have high rates of PTSD from physical or sexual assault, ranging from 30% to 60% in some studies.[129,130] There is also evidence[131] of higher rates of physical and sexual assault among pregnant compared with nonpregnant women. Trauma survivors may use alcohol and drugs to medicate the symptoms of trauma, but often their trauma experience is unrecognized.[132] Trauma-focused interventions for women in substance abuse treatment seem to be safe[133] and may reduce HIV risk.[134] WCDVS (the Women, Co-occurring Disorders and Violence Study)[12,135] reported that integrated services for mental health, substance abuse, and violence in a trauma-informed context are more effective for reducing substance use and improving trauma symptoms and not more costly than treatment as usual. Several trauma-focused therapies for women with co-occurring SUDs have been empirically validated and widely adopted (**Table 7**). These programs focus on establishing safety and support, psychoeducation, and the development of skills and coping strategies for dealing with the effects of trauma and SUDs. See Finkelstein and colleagues[136] for a comprehensive review.

STEPPED CARE ALTERNATIVE TO ASAM PLACEMENT

Handmaker and Wilbourne[146] recommend a stepped care model for intervening with pregnant women who use alcohol and other drugs. Stepped care models represent an alternative to ASAM criterion-base matching and are commonly used in medicine for the treatment of chronic diseases.[16] In stepped care, the lowest intensity and least intrusive level of care is offered first. If that level is not sufficient, then the patient is stepped up to the next highest level (**Fig. 1**). Because many prenatal programs are not equipped with comprehensive and integrated services, stepped care may reduce obstacles faced by pregnant women, such as childcare, transportation, and financial expense.[146] The shift to managed behavioral health care may also have implications for comprehensive and integrated care models, including limiting the range of services available.[147]

Stepped care models may provide more options for pregnant women who are smokers or who meet criteria for alcohol and SUDs but whose problems are characterized as mild, rather than moderate or severe. There is a wide range of substance use patterns among pregnant women, and some may not require residential programs. Prenatal care settings could develop a network of referrals, monitor progress, and make new referrals as necessary to meet the needs of their patients.

In a review and meta-analysis of substance abuse treatment programs for pregnant and parenting women (excluding smoking cessation interventions), Milligan and colleagues[148] determined that integrated (ie, comprehensive services) programs were not significantly more effective in reducing maternal substance use than nonintegrated programs. However, integrated programs did show a small advantage over nonintegrated programs in improving birth outcomes[149] and length of stay.[150] Jansson and colleagues[151] found poorer fetal and birth outcomes for pregnant women who were treated under managed care versus those who received comprehensive care. For women with moderate to severe SUDs and significant psychosocial and psychiatric problems, comprehensive, integrated services in the context of gender-specific (ie, women only) residential or inpatient programs are the treatments of choice.

Table 7
Trauma interventions for women with SUDs

Treatment	Description	Typical Number of Sessions	Manual or Protocol
Helping Women Recover and Beyond Trauma	Combined manual-based treatments for women in criminal justice or correctional settings who have SUD and trauma history Strengths-based approach with focus on safety, coping skills, building healthy relationships and developing a strong interpersonal support network Helping Women Recover has 4 domains: self; relationship/support systems; sexuality; spirituality Beyond Trauma has 3 domains: violence, abuse and trauma; impact of trauma; healing from trauma Community version available for residential and outpatient substance abuse treatment settings	17 recovery plus 11 trauma	Covington SS. Helping women recover: a program for treating addiction[137] Covington SS. Helping women recover: a program for treating substance abuse–Special edition for the criminal justice system[138] Covington SS. A healing journey: a workbook for women[139] Covington SS. Beyond trauma: a healing journey for women. Facilitator's guide[140]
Seeking Safety	Present-focused therapy integrates treatment of both PTSD and substance abuse at the same time Four main content areas: cognitive, behavioral, interpersonal, and case management Safety in relationships, thinking, behavior, and emotions is main goal Group or individual format in outpatient, inpatient, and residential settings	25 (with high degree of flexibility)	Najavits LM. Seeking safety: a treatment manual for PTSD and substance abuse[141] Training Facilitation Guide for Woman's Addiction; available at http://www.seekingsafety.org

Trauma Recovery and Empowerment Model	24–29	Manualized group therapy, gender-specific intervention for women with histories of sexual and physical abuse Draws on cognitive restructuring, psychoeducation, and skills training Emphasizes the development of coping skills and social support Implemented in substance abuse, mental health, and criminal justice settings	Harris M, Community Connections Trauma Work Group. Trauma recovery and empowerment: A clinician's guide for working with women in groups[142] Copeland M, Harris M. Healing the trauma of abuse: A women's workbook[143]
Boston Consortium Model: Trauma-Informed Substance Abuse Treatment for Women	58	Substance abuse and trauma treatment of low-income, minority women Enhanced Trauma Recovery and Empowerment Model with diagnostic assessment and case management Five manual-driven, skills-building group modules (ie, leadership, economics, family reunification, parenting skills)	Amaro H. Protocol for integrating mental health and trauma clinical services into substance abuse treatment[144] Amaro H, McGraw S, Larson MJ, et al. Boston consortium services for families in recovery: A trauma-informed intervention model for women's alcohol and drug addiction treatment[145]

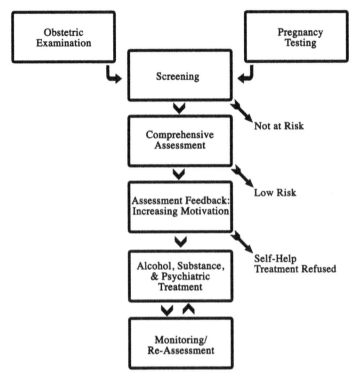

Fig. 1. Stepped care model for intervening with pregnant women who are using alcohol or other substances. (*Adapted from* Handmaker NS, Wilbourne P. Motivational interventions in prenatal clinics. Alcohol Res Health 2001;25(3):228; with permission.)

SUBSTANCE ABUSE TREATMENT SERVICES IN NONTRADITIONAL SETTINGS

The stigma of substance abuse may serve as a barrier for women entering treatment. Low self-esteem, trauma history, responsibility for children, and distrust of providers are among the challenges faced by pregnant women who use substances. Creative and supportive approaches that build on women's strengths should be implemented and studied. One unique harm reduction program in Toronto, Ontario provides comprehensive services (eg, prenatal and postpartum care, case management, pharmacotherapy, addiction treatment, relapse prevention) by an interdisciplinary team for pregnant substance-abusing women in the context of a family medicine setting.[152] This program reported positive maternal and infant health outcomes and suggested that women felt less stigmatized and marginalized obtaining services at a family medicine clinic versus substance abuse treatment program.[153]

EVALUATION AND LONG-TERM RECOMMENDATIONS

There are no safe levels of smoking, alcohol, or drug use during pregnancy. Universal screening, including use of biomarkers when possible, is essential for early identification and intervention with pregnant women. When substance use is identified, a more thorough assessment should be completed to determine scope of treatment needs and appropriate level of care. Programs should match services to the specific needs of each woman and offer a combination of service modalities.[55]

Abstinence or at a minimum harm reduction are important therapeutic goals for pregnant women. SUDs are often (but not always) chronic, relapsing conditions; success can be measured from a variety of perspectives, including time between relapses, duration of abstinence, caring for children, and health care service use.[55] The provider should address substance use in a supportive, empathetic style that promotes patient engagement and acceptance. If a pregnant woman is able to consider using self-help materials, referral to mutual help groups or more structured treatment, this can be an important first step. Provider follow-up, keeping the patient in contact with systems of care and increasing motivation for change, may facilitate treatment entry.

Gender-specific, private and public, outpatient, and residential substance abuse treatment programs have been developed to better meet the specialized needs of substance-abusing pregnant women. However, these services remain limited and reach only a small percentage of women in need of care. For example, in 2011, one-third of US treatment programs had services specifically designed for adult women, and only 13% had services for pregnant or postpartum women.[154] Further, only 36% offered specialized services for clients with co-occurring mental and substance abuse disorders, despite the high rates of comorbid disorders among patients receiving treatment for substance abuse. Clearly, there is a considerable need for expanded access to interventions with proven effectiveness. Additional research is urgently called for to examine evidence-based substance abuse counseling approaches specifically in pregnant and postpartum women. Treatment recommendations are often based on studies with predominantly male samples, thus limiting the strength of our evidence.

There is also increasing research on the usefulness of substance abuse treatment delivery in traditional health care settings, including primary and specialty care clinics. Efforts to colocate substance abuse outpatient care in the obstetrics and gynecology setting may create new opportunities to expand access to and retention in services. Interdisciplinary coordination, in which providers use communication strategies to prevent disruption of services, is critical.

Overall, there is strong evidence that pregnancy may positively influence a woman's motivation for change and acceptance of intervention. Health care providers have an important and influential role in identification of need and guidance toward appropriate care.

REFERENCES

1. American Society of Addiction Medicine. Public policy statement on women, alcohol and other drugs, and pregnancy. Chevy Chase (MD): American Society of Additiction Medicine; 2011.
2. American College of Obstetricians and Gynecologists Committee on Health Care for Underserved Women. Substance abuse reporting and pregnancy: the role of the obstetrician-gynecologist. Committee Opinion No. 473. Obstet Gynecol 2011;117:200–1.
3. Substance Abuse and Mental Health Services Administration. Results from the 2012 National Survey on Drug Use and Health: summary of national findings. NSDUH Series H-46, HHS Publication No. (SMA) 13–4795. Rockville (MD): Substance Abuse and Mental Health Services Administration; 2013.
4. Substance Abuse and Mental Health Services Administration. Results from the 2010 National Survey on Drug Use and Health: summary of national findings. NSDUH Series H-41, HHS Publication No. (SMA) 11–4658. Rockville (MD): Substance Abuse and Mental Health Services Administration; 2011.

5. Tzilos G, Hess L, Kao JC, et al. Characteristics of perinatal women seeking treatment for marijuana abuse in a community-based clinic. Arch Womens Ment Health 2013;16(4):333–7.
6. Jaques SC, Kingsbury A, Henshcke P, et al. Cannabis, the pregnant woman and her child: weeding out the myths. J Perinatol 2014. [Epub ahead of print].
7. Kellogg A, Rose CH, Harms RH, et al. Current trends in narcotic use in pregnancy and neonatal outcomes. Am J Obstet Gynecol 2011;204(3):259.e1–4.
8. Epstein RA, Bobo WV, Martin PR, et al. Increasing pregnancy-related use of prescribed opioid analgesics. Ann Epidemiol 2013;23(8):498–503.
9. Wouldes TA, LaGasse LL, Derauf C, et al. Co-morbidity of substance use disorder and psychopathology in women who use methamphetamine during pregnancy in the US and New Zealand. Drug Alcohol Depend 2013;127(1–3):101–7.
10. Chander G, McCaul ME. Co-occurring psychiatric disorders in women with addictions. Obstet Gynecol Clin North Am 2003;30(3):469–81.
11. Ashley OS, Marsden ME, Brady TM. Effectiveness of substance abuse treatment programming for women: a review. Am J Drug Alcohol Abuse 2003;29(1):19–53.
12. Center for Substance Abuse Treatment. Substance abuse treatment: addressing the specific needs of women. Treatment improvement protocol (TIP) series 51. DHHS Publication No. (SMA) 09–4426. Rockville (MD): Substance Abuse and Mental Health Services Administration; 2009.
13. Center for Substance Abuse Treatment. Substance abuse treatment for persons with co-occurring disorders. Treatment improvement protocol (TIP) series 42. DHHS Publication No. (SMA) 05–3992. Rockville (MD): Substance Abuse and Mental Health Services Administration; 2005.
14. Grella CE. Services for perinatal women with substance abuse and mental health disorders: the unmet need. J Psychoactive Drugs 1997;29(1):67–78.
15. McKetin R, Hickey K, Devlin K, et al. The risk of psychotic symptoms associated with recreational methamphetamine use. Drug Alcohol Rev 2010;29(4):358–63.
16. Miller WR, Forcehimes AA, Zweben A. Treating addiction: a guide for professionals. New York: Guilford Press; 2011.
17. Goler NC, Armstrong MA, Taillac CJ, et al. Substance abuse treatment linked with prenatal visits improves perinatal outcomes: a new standard. J Perinatol 2008;28(9):597–603.
18. Thornberry J, Bhaskar B, Krulewitch CJ, et al. Audio computerized self-report interview use in prenatal clinics. Comput Inform Nurs 2002;20(2):46–52.
19. Fiore M. Treating tobacco use and dependence: 2008 update: clinical practice guideline. Darby (PA): DIANE Publishing; 2008.
20. Russell M, Czarnecki DM, Cowan R, et al. Measures of maternal alcohol use as predictors of development in early childhood. Alcohol Clin Exp Res 1991;15(6):991–1000.
21. Sokol RJ, Martier SS, Ager JW. The T-ACE questions: practical prenatal detection of risk-drinking. Am J Obstet Gynecol 1989;160(4):863–8 [discussion: 8–70].
22. Morse BA, Gehshan S, Hutchins E. Screening for substance abuse during pregnancy: improving care, improving health. Arlington (VA): National Center for Education in Maternal and Child Health; 1997.
23. Ewing H. A practical guide to intervention in health and social services, with pregnant and postpartum addicts and alcoholics. Martinez (CA): The Born Free Project, Contra Costa County Department of Health Services; 1990.
24. Chasnoff IJ, Neuman K, Thornton C, et al. Screening for substance use in pregnancy: a practical approach for the primary care physician. Am J Obstet Gynecol 2001;184(4):752–8.

25. Gaalema DE, Higgins ST, Pepin CS, et al. Illicit drug use among pregnant women enrolled in treatment for cigarette smoking cessation. Nicotine Tob Res 2013;15(5):987–91.

26. Coleman-Cowger VH, Dennis ML, Funk RR, et al. Comparison of the Addiction Severity Index (ASI) and the Global Appraisal of Individual Needs (GAIN) in predicting the effectiveness of drug treatment programs for pregnant and postpartum women. J Subst Abuse Treat 2013;44(1):34–41.

27. McLellan AT, Luborsky L, Woody GE, et al. An improved diagnostic evaluation instrument for substance abuse patients. The Addiction Severity Index. J Nerv Ment Dis 1980;168(1):26–33.

28. Dennis ML, Titus JC, White MK, et al. Global appraisal of individual needs: administration guide for the GAIN and related measures. Bloomington (IL): Chestnut Health Systems; 2003.

29. Spitzer RL, Kroenke K, Williams JB. Validation and utility of a self-report version of PRIME-MD: the PHQ primary care study. Primary Care Evaluation of Mental Disorders. Patient Health Questionnaire. JAMA 1999;282(18): 1737–44.

30. Kelly RH, Zatzick DF, Anders TF. The detection and treatment of psychiatric disorders and substance use among pregnant women cared for in obstetrics. Am J Psychiatry 2001;158(2):213–9.

31. Sheehan DV, Lecrubier Y, Sheehan KH, et al. The validity of the Mini International Neuropsychiatric Interview (MINI) according to the SCID-P and its reliability. Eur Psychiatry 1997;12(5):232–41.

32. Sheehan DV, Lecrubier Y, Sheehan KH, et al. The Mini-International Neuropsychiatric Interview (MINI): the development and validation of a structured diagnostic psychiatric interview for DSM-IV and ICD-10. J Clin Psychiatry 1998; 59(Suppl 20):22–57.

33. Benningfield MM, Dietrich MS, Jones HE, et al. Opioid dependence during pregnancy: relationships of anxiety and depression symptoms to treatment outcomes. Addiction 2012;107(Suppl 1):74–82.

34. Yonkers KA, Forray A, Howell HB, et al. Motivational enhancement therapy coupled with cognitive behavioral therapy versus brief advice: a randomized trial for treatment of hazardous substance use in pregnancy and after delivery. Gen Hosp Psychiatry 2012;34(5):439–49.

35. Substance Abuse and Mental Health Services Administration. Screening, brief intervention and referral to treatment (SBIRT) in behavioral healthcare. Rockville (MD): Substance Abuse and Mental Health Services Administration; 2008.

36. American College of Obstetricians and Gynecologists. At-risk drinking and illicit drug use: ethical issues in obstetric and gynecologic practice. Committee Opinion No 422. Obstet Gynecol 2008;112(6):1449.

37. Peterson L, Gable S, Saldana L. Treatment of maternal addiction to prevent child abuse and neglect. Addict Behav 1996;21(6):789–801.

38. Chamberlain C, O'Mara-Eves A, Oliver S, et al. Psychosocial interventions for supporting women to stop smoking in pregnancy. Cochrane Database Syst Rev 2013;(10):CD001055.

39. Stotts AL, DeLaune KA, Schmitz JM, et al. Impact of a motivational intervention on mechanisms of change in low-income pregnant smokers. Addict Behav 2004;29(8):1649–57.

40. Bullock L, Everett KD, Mullen PD, et al. Baby BEEP: a randomized controlled trial of nurses' individualized social support for poor rural pregnant smokers. Matern Child Health J 2009;13(3):395–406.

41. Cinciripini PM, Blalock JA, Minnix JA, et al. Effects of an intensive depression-focused intervention for smoking cessation in pregnancy. J Consult Clin Psychol 2010;78(1):44–54.
42. Naughton F, Prevost AT, Sutton S. Self-help smoking cessation interventions in pregnancy: a systematic review and meta-analysis. Addiction 2008;103(4):566–79.
43. Valbo A, Eide T. Smoking cessation in pregnancy: the effect of hypnosis in a randomized study. Addict Behav 1996;21(1):29–35.
44. Cope GF, Nayyar P, Holder R. Feedback from a point-of-care test for nicotine intake to reduce smoking during pregnancy. Ann Clin Biochem 2003;40(Pt 6):674–9.
45. Tuten M, Fitzsimons H, Chisolm MS, et al. Contingent incentives reduce cigarette smoking among pregnant, methadone-maintained women: results of an initial feasibility and efficacy randomized clinical trial. Addiction 2012;107(10):1868–77.
46. Donatelle RJ, Prows SL, Champeau D, et al. Randomised controlled trial using social support and financial incentives for high risk pregnant smokers: Significant Other Supporter (SOS) program. Tob Control 2000;9:67–9.
47. Heil SH, Higgins ST, Bernstein IM, et al. Effects of voucher-based incentives on abstinence from cigarette smoking and fetal growth among pregnant women. Addiction 2008;103(6):1009–18.
48. Higgins ST, Washio Y, Heil SH, et al. Financial incentives for smoking cessation among pregnant and newly postpartum women. Prev Med 2012;55(Suppl):S33–40.
49. Flemming K, Graham H, Heirs M, et al. Smoking in pregnancy: a systematic review of qualitative research of women who commence pregnancy as smokers. J Adv Nurs 2013;69(5):1023–36.
50. Stade BC, Bailey C, Dzendoletas D, et al. Psychological and/or educational interventions for reducing alcohol consumption in pregnant women and women planning pregnancy. Cochrane Database Syst Rev 2009;(2):CD004228.
51. Gilinsky A, Swanson V, Power K. Interventions delivered during antenatal care to reduce alcohol consumption during pregnancy: a systematic review. Addict Res Theory 2011;19(3):235–50.
52. O'Connor MJ, Whaley SE. Brief intervention for alcohol use by pregnant women. Am J Public Health 2007;97(2):252–8.
53. Chang G, McNamara TK, Orav EJ, et al. Brief intervention for prenatal alcohol use: a randomized trial. Obstet Gynecol Annu 2005;105(5):991–8.
54. Reynolds KD, Coombs DW, Lowe JB, et al. Evaluation of a self-help program to reduce alcohol consumption among pregnant women. Int J Addict 1995;30(4):427–43.
55. Howell EM, Chasnoff IJ. Perinatal substance abuse treatment. Findings from focus groups with clients and providers. J Subst Abuse Treat 1999;17(1–2):139–48.
56. Bell K, Cramer-Benjamin D, Anastas J. Predicting length of stay of substance-using pregnant and postpartum women in day treatment. J Subst Abuse Treat 1997;14(4):393–400.
57. Smith IE, Dent DZ, Coles CD, et al. A comparison study of treated and untreated pregnant and postpartum cocaine-abusing women. J Subst Abuse Treat 1992;9(4):343–8.
58. Miller WR, Rollnick S. Motivational interviewing: helping people change. 3rd edition. New York: Guilford Press; 2012.

59. Nowinski J, Baker S. The twelve step facilitation handbook: a systematic approach to recovery from substance dependence. The project MATCH twelve step treatment protocol. Center City (MN): Hazelden Foundation; 2006.
60. Schottenfeld RS, Moore B, Pantalon MV. Contingency management with community reinforcement approach or twelve-step facilitation drug counseling for cocaine dependent pregnant women or women with young children. Drug Alcohol Depend 2011;118(1):48–55.
61. Moos RH, Moos BS, Timko C. Gender, treatment and self-help in remission from alcohol use disorders. Clin Med Res 2006;4(3):163–74.
62. Kadden R, Carroll K, Donovan D, et al. Cognitive-behavioral coping skills therapy manual: a clinical research guide for therapists treating individuals with alcohol abuse and dependence (NIH Publication No. 94–3727). Rockville (MD): National Institutes of Health, National Institute on Alcohol Abuse and Alcoholism; 2003.
63. Sobell LC, Sobell MB. Group therapy for substance use disorders: a motivational cognitive-behavioral approach. New York: Guilford Press; 2011.
64. Burns A, O Mahen H, Baxter H, et al. A pilot randomised controlled trial of cognitive behavioural therapy for antenatal depression. BMC Psychiatry 2013; 13(1):33.
65. O'Mahen H, Himle JA, Fedock G, et al. A pilot randomized controlled trial of cognitive behavioral therapy for perinatal depression adapted for women with low incomes. Depress Anxiety 2013;30(7):679–87.
66. Miller WR, Zweben A, Diclemente C, et al. Motivational enhancement therapy: a clinical research guide for therapists treating individuals with alcohol abuse and dependence (NIH Publication No. 94–3723). Rockville (MD): National Institutes of Health, National Institute on Alcohol Abuse and Alcoholism; 1994.
67. Miller WR. Motivational enhancement therapy with drug abusers. Albuquerque (NM): University of New Mexico, Department of Psychology and Center on Alcoholism, Substance Abuse, and Addictions; 1995.
68. Petry NM, Stitzer M. Contingency management: using motivational incentives to improve drug abuse treatment. West Haven (CT): Yale University Psychotherapy Development Center; 2002.
69. Petry NM. Contingency management for substance abuse treatment: a guide to implementing this evidence-based practice. New York: Routledge; 2012.
70. O'Farrell T, Fals-Stewart T. Behavioral couples therapy for alcoholism and drug abuse. New York: Guilford Press; 2006.
71. Fals-Stewart T, O'Farrell T, Birchler G, et al. Behavioral couples therapy for drug abuse and alcoholism: a 12 step manual. 2nd edition. Buffalo (NY): Addiction and Family Research Group; 2006.
72. Fals-Stewart W, Birchler GR, Kelley ML. Learning sobriety together: a randomized clinical trial examining behavioral couples therapy with alcoholic female patients. J Consult Clin Psychol 2006;74(3):579–91.
73. Winters J, Fals-Stewart W, O'Farrell TJ, et al. Behavioral couples therapy for female substance-abusing patients: effects on substance use and relationship adjustment. J Consult Clin Psychol 2002;70(2):344–55.
74. McCrady BS, Epstein EE, Cook S, et al. A randomized trial of individual and couple behavioral alcohol treatment for women. J Consult Clin Psychol 2009; 77(2):243–56.
75. Schumm JA, O'Farrell TJ, Murphy CM, et al. Partner violence before and after couples-based alcoholism treatment for female alcoholic patients. J Consult Clin Psychol 2009;77(6):1136–46.

76. Handmaker NS, Miller WR, Manicke M. Findings of a pilot study of motivational interviewing with pregnant drinkers. J Stud Alcohol Drugs 1999;60(2):285–7.

77. Osterman RL, Dyehouse J. Effects of a motivational interviewing intervention to decrease prenatal alcohol use. West J Nurs Res 2012;34(4):434–54.

78. Stotts AL, Diclemente CC, Dolan-Mullen P. One-to-one: a motivational intervention for resistant pregnant smokers. Addict Behav 2002;27(2):275–92.

79. Haug NA, Svikis DS, Diclemente C. Motivational enhancement therapy for nicotine dependence in methadone-maintained pregnant women. Psychol Addict Behav 2004;18(3):289–92.

80. Ershoff DH, Quinn VP, Boyd NR, et al. The Kaiser Permanente prenatal smoking-cessation trial. Am J Prev Med 1999;17(3):161–8.

81. Tappin DM, Lumsden MA, Gilmour WH, et al. Randomised controlled trial of home based motivational interviewing by midwives to help pregnant smokers quit or cut down. BMJ 2005;331(7513):373–7.

82. Hayes CB, Collins C, O'Carroll H, et al. Effectiveness of motivational interviewing in influencing smoking cessation in pregnant and postpartum disadvantaged women. Nicotine Tob Res 2013;15(5):969–77.

83. Winhusen T, Somoza E, Ciraulo DA, et al. A double-blind, placebo-controlled trial of tiagabine for the treatment of cocaine dependence. Drug Alcohol Depend 2007;91(2–3):141–8.

84. Terplan M, Lui S. Psychosocial interventions for pregnant women in outpatient illicit drug treatment programs compared to other interventions. Cochrane Database Syst Rev 2007;(4):CD006037.

85. Hull L, May J, Farrell-Moore D, et al. Treatment of cocaine abuse during pregnancy: translating research to clinical practice. Curr Psychiatry Rep 2010; 12(5):454–61.

86. Prendergast M, Podus D, Finney J, et al. Contingency management for treatment of substance use disorders: a meta-analysis. Addiction 2006;101(11): 1546–60.

87. McCaul ME, Svikis DS. Measures of service utilization. In: Rahdert ER, editor. Treatment for drug-exposed women and children: advances in research methodology, vol. 166. Rockville (MD): National Institute on Drug Abuse; 1996. p. 225–41.

88. Jones HE, Haug N, Silverman K, et al. The effectiveness of incentives in enhancing treatment attendance and drug abstinence in methadone-maintained pregnant women. Drug Alcohol Depend 2001;61(3):297–306.

89. Elk R, Mangus L, Rhoades H, et al. Cessation of cocaine use during pregnancy: effects of contingency management interventions on maintaining abstinence and complying with prenatal care. Addict Behav 1998;23(1):57–64.

90. Elk R, Schmitz J, Spiga R, et al. Behavioral treatment of cocaine-dependent pregnant women and TB-exposed patients. Addict Behav 1995;20(4):533–42.

91. Tuten M, Svikis DS, Keyser-Marcus L, et al. Lessons learned from a randomized trial of fixed and escalating contingency management schedules in opioid-dependent pregnant women. Am J Drug Alcohol Abuse 2012;38(4):286–92.

92. Laken M, McComish J, Ager J. Predictors of prenatal substance use and birth weight during outpatient treatment. J Subst Abuse Treat 1997;14(4):359–66.

93. Marsh JC, Smith BD. Integrated substance abuse and child welfare services for women: a progress review. Child Youth Serv Rev 2011;33(3):466–72.

94. Center for Substance Abuse Treatment. Substance abuse: clinical issues in intensive outpatient treatment. Treatment improvement protocol (TIP) series 47. DHHS Publication No. (SMA) 06–4182. Rockville (MD): Substance Abuse and Mental Health Services Administration; 2006.

95. Center for Substance Abuse Treatment. Counselor's treatment manual: matrix intensive outpatient treatment for people with stimulant use disorders. DHHS Publication No. (SMA) 06–4152. Rockville (MD): Center for Substance Abuse Treatment. Substance Abuse and Mental Health Services Administration; 2006.

96. Strantz IH, Welch SP. Postpartum women in outpatient drug abuse treatment: correlates of retention/completion. J Psychoactive Drugs 1995;27(4):357–73.

97. Jones HE, O'Grady KE, Tuten M. Reinforcement-based treatment improves the maternal treatment and neonatal outcomes of pregnant patients enrolled in comprehensive care treatment. Am J Addict 2011;20(3):196–204.

98. Conners NA, Grant A, Crone CC, et al. Substance abuse treatment for mothers: treatment outcomes and the impact of length of stay. J Subst Abuse Treat 2006; 31(4):447–56.

99. Greenfield L, Burgdorf K, Chen X, et al. Effectiveness of long-term residential substance abuse treatment for women: findings from three national studies. Am J Drug Alcohol Abuse 2004;30(3):537–50.

100. De Leon G, Jainchill N, Bull NY. Residential therapeutic communities for female substance abusers. Acad Med 1991;67(3):277–90.

101. Comfort M, Kaltenbach KA. Biopsychosocial characteristics and treatment outcomes of pregnant cocaine-dependent women in residential and outpatient substance abuse treatment. J Psychoactive Drugs 1999;31(3):279–89.

102. Burgdorf K, Dowell K, Chen XW, et al. Birth outcomes for pregnant women in residential substance abuse treatment. Eval Program Plann 2004;27(2): 199–204.

103. Svikis DS, Golden AS, Huggins GR, et al. Cost-effectiveness of treatment for drug-abusing pregnant women. Drug Alcohol Depend 1997;45(1–2):105–13.

104. Center for Substance Abuse Treatment. Therapeutic community curriculum: participant's manual. DHHS publication no. (SMA) 06-4122. Rockville (MD): Center for Substance Abuse Treatment. Substance Abuse and Mental Health Services Administration; 2006.

105. De Leon G. The therapeutic community: theory, model, and method. New York: Springer; 2000.

106. Condelli WS, Koch MA, Fletcher B. Treatment refusal/attrition among adults randomly assigned to programs at a drug treatment campus–the New Jersey Substance Abuse Treatment Campus, Seacaucus, NJ. J Subst Abuse Treat 2000;18(4):395–407.

107. Sacks S, De Leon G, Bernhardt A, et al. Modified therapeutic community for homeless mentally ill chemical abusers: treatment manual. New York: National Development and Research Institutes/Center for Therapeutic Community Research; 1996.

108. Sacks SS, Sacks JY, De Leon G. Treatment for MICAs: design and implementation of the modified TC. J Psychoactive Drugs 1999;31(1):19–30.

109. Price A, Simmel C. Partners influence on women's addiction and recovery: the connection between substance abuse, trauma, and intimate relationships. Berkeley (CA): National Abandoned Infants Assistance Resource Center, University of California at Berkeley; 2002.

110. Grella CE. Women in residential drug treatment: differences by program type and pregnancy. J Health Care Poor Underserved 1999;10(2):216–29.

111. Claus RE, Orwin RG, Kissin W, et al. Does gender-specific substance abuse treatment for women promote continuity of care? J Subst Abuse Treat 2007; 32(1):27–39.

112. Hser YI, Maglione M, Polinsky ML, et al. Predicting drug treatment entry among treatment-seeking individuals. J Subst Abuse Treat 1998;15(3):213–20.

113. Chen XW, Burgdorf K, Dowell K, et al. Factors associated with retention of drug abusing women in long-term residential treatment. Eval Program Plann 2004; 27(2):205–12.

114. Hughes PH, Coletti SD, Neri RL, et al. Retaining cocaine-abusing women in a therapeutic community: the effect of a child live-in program. Am J Public Health 1995;85(8 Pt 1):1149–52.

115. Szuster RR, Rich LL, Chung A, et al. Treatment retention in women's residential chemical dependency treatment: the effect of admission with children. Subst Use Misuse 1996;31(8):1001–13.

116. Lundgren LM, Schilling RF, Fitzgerald T, et al. Parental status of women injection drug users and entry to methadone maintenance. Subst Use Misuse 2003;38(8): 1109–31.

117. Saunders EJ. A new model of residential care for substance-abusing women and their children. Adult Residential Care Journal 1993;7(2):104–17.

118. Stevens SJ, Patton T. Residential treatment for drug addicted women and their children: effective treatment strategies. Drugs Soc 1998;13(1–2):235–49.

119. Killeen T, Brady KT. Parental stress and child behavioral outcomes following substance abuse residential treatment. Follow-up at 6 and 12 months. J Subst Abuse Treat 2000;19(1):23–9.

120. Miles DR, Kulstad JL, Haller DL. Severity of substance abuse and psychiatric problems among perinatal drug-dependent women. J Psychoactive Drugs 2002;34(4):339–46.

121. Benningfield MM, Arria AM, Kaltenbach K, et al. Co-occurring psychiatric symptoms are associated with increased psychological, social, and medical impairment in opioid dependent pregnant women. Am J Addict 2010;19(5): 416–21.

122. Fitzsimons HE, Tuten M, Vaidya V, et al. Mood disorders affect drug treatment success of drug-dependent pregnant women. J Subst Abuse Treat 2007; 32(1):19–25.

123. Miles DR, Svikis DS, Kulstad JL, et al. Psychopathology in pregnant drug-dependent women with and without comorbid alcohol dependence. Alcohol Clin Exp Res 2001;25(7):1012–7.

124. Fiocchi FF, Kingree JB. Treatment retention and birth outcomes of crack users enrolled in a substance abuse treatment program for pregnant women. J Subst Abuse Treat 2001;20(2):137–42.

125. Haller DL, Knisely JS, Elswick RK Jr, et al. Perinatal substance abusers: factors influencing treatment retention. J Subst Abuse Treat 1997;14(6):513–9.

126. Tuten M, Heil SH, O'Grady KE, et al. The impact of mood disorders on the delivery and neonatal outcomes of methadone-maintained pregnant patients. Am J Drug Alcohol Abuse 2009;35(5):358–63.

127. Linares Scott TJ, Heil SH, Higgins ST, et al. Depressive symptoms predict smoking status among pregnant women. Addict Behav 2009;34(8):705–8.

128. Lopez WD, Konrath SH, Seng JS. Abuse-related post-traumatic stress, coping, and tobacco use in pregnancy. J Obstet Gynecol Neonatal Nurs 2011;40(4): 422–31.

129. Najavits LM, Weiss RD, Shaw SR. The link between substance abuse and post-traumatic stress disorder in women–a research review. Am J Addict 1997;6(4): 273–83.

130. Ouimette P, Goodwin E, Brown PJ. Health and well being of substance use disorder patients with and without posttraumatic stress disorder. Addict Behav 2006;31(8):1415–23.

131. Burch RL, Gallup GG. Pregnancy as a stimulus for domestic violence. Journal of Family Violence 2004;19(4):243–7.

132. Covington SS, Burke C, Keaton S, et al. Evaluation of a trauma-informed and gender-responsive intervention for women in drug treatment. J Psychoactive Drugs 2008;5(Suppl):387–98.

133. Killeen T, Hien D, Campbell A, et al. Adverse events in an integrated trauma-focused intervention for women in community substance abuse treatment. J Subst Abuse Treat 2008;35(3):304–11.

134. Hien DA, Campbell AN, Killeen T, et al. The impact of trauma-focused group therapy upon HIV sexual risk behaviors in the NIDA Clinical Trials Network "Women and trauma" multi-site study. AIDS Behav 2010;14(2):421–30.

135. Moses DJ, Huntington N, D'Ambrosio B. Developing integrated services for women with co-occurring disorders and trauma histories. Women, Co-Occurring Disorders, and Violence Study. Delmar (NY): Policy Research Associates, Inc; 2004.

136. Finkelstein N, VandeMark N, Fallot R, et al. Enhancing substance abuse recovery through integrated trauma treatment. Sarasota (FL): National Trauma Consortium; 2004.

137. Covington SS. Helping women recover: a program for treating addiction. San Francisco (CA): Jossey-Bass; 2008.

138. Covington SS. Helping women recover: a program for treating substance abuse–special edition for the criminal justice system. San Francisco (CA): Jossey-Bass; 2008.

139. Covington SS. A healing journey: a workbook for women. Center City (MN): Hazelden; 2003.

140. Covington SS. Beyond trauma: a healing journey for women. Facilitator's guide. Center City (MN): Hazelden; 2003.

141. Najavits LM. Seeking safety: a treatment manual for PTSD and substance abuse. New York: Guilford Press; 2002.

142. Harris M, Community Connections Trauma Work Group. Trauma recovery and empowerment: a clinician's guide for working with women in groups. New York: Community Connections; 1998.

143. Copeland M, Harris M. Healing the trauma of abuse: a women's workbook. Oakland (CA): New Harbinger Publications, Inc; 2000.

144. Amaro H. Protocol for integrating mental health and trauma clinical services into substance abuse treatment. Boston: Author; 2009.

145. Amaro H, McGraw S, Larson MJ, et al. Boston consortium services for families in recovery: a trauma-informed intervention model for women's alcohol and drug addiction treatment. Alcohol Treat Q 2004;22(3–4):95–119.

146. Handmaker NS, Wilbourne P. Motivational interventions in prenatal clinics. Alcohol Res Health 2001;25(3):219–29.

147. Galanter M, Keller DS, Dermatis H, et al. The impact of managed care on substance abuse treatment: a report of the American Society of Addiction Medicine. J Addict Dis 2000;19(3):13–34.

148. Milligan K, Niccols A, Sword W, et al. Maternal substance use and integrated treatment programs for women with substance abuse issues and their children: a meta-analysis. Subst Abuse Treat Prev Policy 2010;5:21.

149. Milligan K, Niccols A, Sword W, et al. Birth outcomes for infants born to women participating in integrated substance abuse treatment programs: a meta-analytic review. Addict Res Theory 2011;19(6):542–55.

150. Milligan K, Niccols A, Sword W, et al. Length of stay and treatment completion for mothers with substance abuse issues in integrated treatment programmes. Drugs: Education, Prevention and Policy 2011;18(3):219–27.

151. Jansson LM, Svikis DS, Velez M, et al. The impact of managed care on drug-dependent pregnant and postpartum women and their children. Subst Use Misuse 2007;42(6):961–74.

152. Ordean A, Kahan M. Comprehensive treatment program for pregnant substance users in a family medicine clinic. Can Fam Physician 2011;57(11):e430–5.

153. Lefebvre L, Midmer D, Boyd JA, et al. Participant perception of an integrated program for substance abuse in pregnancy. J Obstet Gynecol Neonatal Nurs 2010;39(1):46–52.

154. Substance Abuse and Mental Health Services Administration. National Survey of Substance Abuse Treatment Services (N-SSATS): 2011 data on substance abuse treatment facilities. BHSIS Series: S-64, HHS publication no. (SMA) 12–4730. Rockville (MD): Substance Abuse and Mental Health Services Administration; 2012.

The Perils of Opioid Prescribing During Pregnancy

Marjorie Meyer, MD

KEYWORDS

• Pregnancy • Opioids • Chronic pain • Teratogens • Neonatal abstinence

KEY POINTS

- Chronic opioid therapy during periconception can result in congenital anomalies.
- Neonates exposed to chronic opioid therapy in utero are at risk for neonatal abstinence symptoms.
- Opioids kept in the home should be secured from children and teens in the household to prevent accidental poisoning or experimentation.
- Chronic opioid therapy during pregnancy requires a multidisciplinary approach with obstetrics, pain specialists, and pediatricians.
- Women planning pregnancy or not using reliable contraception should be on folic acid before conception.

IS PRESCRIBING OPIOIDS FOR CHRONIC PAIN PERILOUS FOR WOMEN?

Prescribing long-term opioid therapy to women has increased dramatically over the last decade, with the incidence of use as high as 10% in reproductive aged women in some health care systems.[1] This statistic makes it hardly surprising that prescribing of opioids during pregnancy has increased in a parallel fashion.[2] Despite limited evidence of efficacy of chronic opioid therapy for the types of pain most commonly reported in women,[3] clinicians will care for patients that become pregnant while taking opioids for chronic pain. The purpose of this article is to examine the perils of chronic opioid use in women in general, during pregnancy, and on the neonate.

RISK FOR MISPRESCRIPTION

Women have more pain than men. Although the cellular mechanisms underlying the sexual dimorphism of pain response remains unclear,[4] epidemiologic studies are consistent in the finding of increased chronic pain syndromes in women.[5] Women

No financial disclosures.
Fletcher Allen Health Care and the University of Vermont, 111 Colchester Avenue, Burlington, VT 05401, USA
E-mail address: Marjorie.meyer@uvm.edu

Obstet Gynecol Clin N Am 41 (2014) 297–306
http://dx.doi.org/10.1016/j.ogc.2014.02.006
0889-8545/14/$ – see front matter © 2014 Elsevier Inc. All rights reserved.

obgyn.theclinics.com

receive more opioid prescriptions than men, have chronic use more frequently, and are prescribed higher doses.[3,6] A recent review by Darnall and colleagues[3] details the evidence available for common indications for opioid treatment in women. There is no evidence to support long-term opioid use for irritable bowel symptoms, headache, or fibromyalgia, and at best, mixed evidence of efficacy for musculoskeletal pain. Once opioid use has exceeded 90 days, two-thirds of patients are still taking these drugs years later.[7] Preexisting depression, anxiety, and smoking increase the risk of long-term opioid prescribing.[3] Of women entering a treatment program for prescription drug abuse, 62% received the initial prescription legitimately by a physician (as opposed to illegally); over half continued opioid use through legitimate prescription, but were more than twice as likely as men to have multiple prescribers.[8,9] Women who abuse prescription opioids are less likely to use opioids through a route other than orally (ie, less intravenous [IV] or intranasal use compared to men), but are more likely to use medication to modulate negative effect and psychiatric symptoms, as opposed to pain. Although some investigators suggest that opioids may play a role in the treatment of long-term multimodality pain and suffering,[7] this approach has not been rigorously tested or accepted and would be beyond the scope of the general practitioner.

Overall, these findings suggest that opioids prescribed by well-intentioned providers for poorly defined pain sets the stage for chronic, higher dose opioid use for modulation of negative effect, taking a toll on the women's life and family.[8,9]

RISK FOR MISUSE, ADDICTION, OR DEPENDENCE

The blurry lines between misuse, physical dependence, and addition have been simplified in the most recent Diagnostic and Statistical Manual of the American Psychiatric Association fifth edition.[10] Physical dependence has been defined as a state of adaptation that is manifested by a drug class–specific withdrawal syndrome produced by abrupt cessation, rapid dose reduction, decreasing blood level of the drug, and/or administration of an antagonist.[11] Historically, the physical symptoms associated with cessation of a drug (physical withdrawal) were differentiated from substance addiction or dependence, with the latter characterized by a specific preoccupation with a desire to obtain and take the drug and persistent drug-seeking behavior. The various definitions of dependence and addiction can explain why the prevalence of addiction in individuals prescribed opioids for long periods of time ranges from 0% to 50%. In the most recent DSM-5 substance use disorder, these characteristics have been combined. Regardless of definition, there is no evidence that women are more prone to misuse, dependence, or addition than men who are prescribed long-term opioid therapy; however, it is clear that for women seeking treatment for misuse, the negative impact on family, social life, and employment is greater than men with similar medical functional impairment.[8,9] Hence, another peril of prescribing chronic opioids to women: the sequelae of dependence or misuse are more severe than for men.

RISK FOR OVERDOSE

Between 1999 and 2007, the risk for unintentional opioid overdose–related death has increased by 124%.[12] Although men are more likely to die following an opioid-related overdose, hospitalization following prescription drug overdose has been higher for women (2009: 16,000/100, 000) than men (2009: 13,000/100000) since 1993 and escalating more rapidly.[6,13] In a predominantly male cohort,[12] there is a relationship between the dose and manner in which opioids are prescribed and the risk for opioid-related overdose death: the hazard ratio (HR) for opioid-related overdose death for individuals prescribed a maximum of 100 mg/d or more (morphine equivalents, compared to 1–20 mg/d) was increased among those with chronic pain (HR) 7.18 (95% confidence interval [CI], 4.85–10.65, absolute risk difference approximation 0.25%) and with substance use disorders (HR) 4.54 (95% CI, 2.46–8.37; absolute risk difference approximation 0.14%). There is ample evidence that prescribing for women is equally perilous. In 2010, prescription opioids were involved in 71.3% of the 9292 prescription drug–specified deaths among women, a 41.5% increase from 1999.[6] Age and race factor into the risk of prescription opioid–related death, with the death of women in reproductive age increasing approximately 125% and American/Indian and non-Hispanic white women at highest risk. Finally, there has been a dramatic increase in heroin-related overdose since 2007, especially in the 20 to 24 year age bracket. Although a causal link cannot be made between the increase in prescription drug use and new onset heroin use, it is consistent with population dynamic models.[13] Half of the pregnancy-associated nonnatural death that occurred in Florida between 1999 and 2005 involved prescription opioids alone or in combination with other drugs.[14] Together, these data highlight another peril of opioid prescribing: it can be fatal.

RISK TO CHILDREN AND ADOLESCENTS

The presence of opioid prescriptions poses a risk to others in the home, particularly small children and adolescents. Adult medication prescriptions are significantly associated with exposures and poisonings of children of all ages.[15] There has been an increase in childhood opioid poisoning mirroring the increase in adult opioid overdose,[13,15] with a 27% risk of severe injury or 35% risk of hospitalization following opioid exposure. From 2006 to 2009, adult use of prescription opioids increased from about 3% to about 7% from 2006 to 2009; for every 1% increase in adults taking opioids there was an increase in the poisoning of 1.5/million children aged 0 to 5 years, despite recent changes in packaging.[15]

For younger children, exposure tends to be related to exploratory behavior with unintentional use. Among teens, ingestion is more likely to be intentional, with the intention for recreation or self-harm. Teen exposures are associated with substantial risk, with 40% of emergency room visits for opioid exposure among 13 to 19 year olds requiring admission to the hospital, compared with 14% of visits among 0 to 5 year olds. The number of emergency visits involving nonmedical use of opioid prescriptions more than doubled from 2004 to 2008 for patients younger than 21 years old.[16] More than one-third of these patients using nonmedical use of opioid prescriptions obtained these medications from leftover prescriptions of their own and over half received the opioid for free from a friend or relative. Among high school seniors, there was more nonmedical use of opioids from a previous prescription among women compared with men (42% vs 31%). When young injection drug users were asked about initial exposure, a third reported first exposure with prescription opioids pilfered from a family member's prescription.[17] These data outline the collateral damage of opioid prescribing: medication in the home risks accidental use by children or intentional misuse by adolescents, with disastrous long-term consequences.

RISKS OF PRESCRIBING BEFORE PREGNANCY (PERICONCEPTION)

The risk for unintended pregnancy in the United States is almost 50%, increasing to almost 90% for women with opioid dependence.[18,19] For women not using long-acting contraception, the perils of opioid use in early pregnancy should be discussed.

First trimester opioid exposure occurs in 2% to 3% of pregnancies.[20] The largest population-based study was performed by Broussard, using the population studied in the National Birth Defects Prevention Study from 1997 to 2005. Women having a child with a birth defect and control women were interviewed about medication habits from 1 month before 3 months after conception. This study found that women who used opioids during this time frame had an increased risk for fetal cardiac defects, particularly conoventricular septal defects (odds ratio [OR] 2.7; 95% CI, 1.1–6.3); hypoplastic left heart syndrome (OR 2.4; 95% CI, 1.4–4.1), neural tube defects (OR 2.0; 95% CI, 1.3–3.2), or gastroschisis (OR 1.8, 95% CI, 1.1–2.9). A separate study based in Washington state reported the association of early pregnancy opioid exposure and open neural tube defects (OR 2.2, 95% CI, 1.2–4.2). Despite the limitations of these studies—recall bias and lack of information regarding the indication for opioid treatment—the teratogenic risk of opioids should be discussed with women considering long-term opioids to manage pain. The addition of teratogen warnings to all opioid prescriptions has been suggested but has not been initiated.[21] Preconceptional folic acid (0.8 mg or higher) can reduce the incidence of neural tube defects, with more recent evidence suggesting reductions in cardiac defects and low birthweight.[22,23] Women of reproductive age not using long-acting contraception should receive folic acid supplementation; whether this can decrease opioid-related congenital anomalies is unknown.

RISKS OF PRESCRIBING DURING PREGNANCY/POST PARTUM

The prevalence of opioid prescribing during pregnancy has increased over the last 10 years.[2,24] In Tennessee, the number of opioid prescriptions increased 37% from 268 to 368/1000 pregnancies; 29% of women filled a prescription for opioids during pregnancy, with a median duration of 4 days, suggesting acute pain as the primary indication.[24] In Minnesota, the rate of narcotic use for more than 1 month during pregnancy increased from 1/1000 to 5/1000 deliveries.[2]

The data regarding outcomes of pregnancies in which opioids have been prescribed for chronic pain, as opposed to treatment of opioid dependence, are limited. The most serious risk to neonates exposed to opioids during pregnancy due to chronic pain is iatrogenic late preterm birth or early term birth. Kellog[2] reported on neonatal admission to the intensive care unit for neonates exposed to narcotics during pregnancy: 72/177 (41%) infants required admission to the neonatal intensive care unit, mostly for complications of early term delivery such as respiratory complications, hypoglycemia, jaundice, and difficulty feeding; only 10/177 infants (5.6%) were admitted for neonatal abstinence symptoms. When comparing neonatal outcome of pregnancies treated for chronic pain versus for opioid dependence, Sharpe[25] found the median gestational age in those infants exposed to opioids for chronic pain 2 weeks shorter for those treated for opioid dependence (gestational age 37 weeks vs 39 weeks); 11/19 (58%) neonates in the pain group were preterm as opposed to 3/24 (13%) neonates exposed to opioids for maternal opioid addiction. Infants of mothers treated for chronic pain were larger (after correction for earlier gestational age) and required treatment of neonatal abstinence less frequently (chronic pain: 11%; opioid dependence 58%).

In summary, there are perils to the neonate exposed to chronic opioid therapy during pregnancy: iatrogenic early delivery for maternal pain increases the risk for neonatal morbidity. The risk for neonatal abstinence symptoms is lower than that observed for neonates exposed to opioids for the treatment of opioid addiction and is quite reassuring, although postnatal evaluation for neonatal abstinence symptoms is still required.

Breastfeeding when mothers are prescribed short-acting opioids for acute, puerperal pain has been standard practice for years. The death of a breastfed neonate attributed to maternal codeine ingestion was reported in 2006.[26] This mother was found to have a duplication of the cytochrome p450 2d6 gene, which resulted in ultra-rapid conversion of codeine to morphine (the active metabolite) with high breast milk concentration of morphine. In 2007, the Food and Drug Administration issued a warning about the use of codeine and breastfeeding following reports of life-threatening sedation in breastfeeding infants. Although oxycodone was considered an alternative, sedation with either codeine or oxycodone was observed in almost 20% of breastfeeding infants when opioid-naïve mothers are treated for postpartum pain, compared with only 0.5% of breastfed neonates of mothers taking only acetaminophen.[27] There is concern that these adverse events are more common than reported as they are poorly captured by national reporting mechanisms.[28]

It is not known whether infants of mothers taking short-acting opioids chronically during pregnancy are at a similar risk for sedation with breastfeeding. Because these infants are at risk for neonatal abstinence symptoms, they may be more tolerant to opioids and less susceptible to sedation from breast milk exposure, although this has not been demonstrated. This concept is supported by the finding that maternal somnolence from opioids correlates with neonatal sedation,[27] as does maternal dose and duration of treatment. Nonetheless, there are alternatives to codeine for pain control following delivery, and avoidance would be prudent. When either codeine or oxycodone is prescribed to breastfeeding women, the mother and neonate should be monitored for sedation.[29]

In summary, chronic opioid therapy during pregnancy poses unique risks to the pregnancy and neonate: iatrogenic prematurity and neonatal somnolence with breastfeeding, in addition to the well-described neonatal abstinence symptoms.

WHY OPIOIDS + SMOKING IS PARTICULARLY PERILOUS

Studies are remarkably consistent in the finding that smokers, in general, are more likely to require chronic opioid therapy for pain, require higher doses of opioids for pain control, have a higher risk of drug dependence, and exhibit more aberrant drug-taking behaviors compared to nonsmokers. Risks were uniformly greater in those individuals smoking more than 1 pack per day.[30] During pregnancy, smoking poses the additional concerns of poor fetal growth, abruption, stillbirth, and preterm birth.

Risk for concurrent use of smoking and opioids is not limited to maternal opioid dependence and pregnancy complications. Infants exhibiting neonatal abstinence symptoms after in utero exposure to methadone or buprenorphine for treatment of opioid dependence had increasing neonatal abstinence symptoms and duration of treatment of abstinence symptoms with increasing maternal smoking.[31]

Reduction of smoking volume during pregnancy can improve fetal growth, even if cessation cannot be achieved.[32] Patients maintained on opioids for chronic pain should be aware that smoking increases risk for any pregnancy and may increase neonatal abstinence symptoms.

HOW TO APPROACH THE PREGNANT PATIENT ON CHRONIC OPIOID THERAPY FOR PAIN

Despite the increase in the prevalence of opioid use in pregnancy, the data regarding pregnancy and neonatal outcomes for women treated with opioids for chronic pain during pregnancy remain limited. An understanding of the underlying disease requiring chronic opioid use for pain and optimization of treatment is an obvious first step (**Box 1**). An exploration regarding alternatives for pain control should be revisited in the context of pregnancy, as the patient may reconsider risk/benefit of continued opioid use. A good place to start would be revisiting the patient/selection and risk stratification in the Guidelines for use of chronic opioid therapy.[33] The optimal candidate has moderate to severe pain, has failed other modalities, has improved function with opioid therapy, and does not have a history or drug or alcohol abuse. A fresh assessment of current pain and therapeutic efficacy of chronic opioids, in the context of pregnancy, is warranted. Excellent communication between the provider prescribing opioids and the obstetric provider is essential, with appropriate Health Insurance Probability and Accountability Act consents to allow free information exchange. Providers should decide who will prescribe during pregnancy, assess for therapeutic goals, and develop a plan for pain escalations during pregnancy. Random urine drug screens should be routinely performed for patients with a history of illicit use and considered for patients without such history. Although treatment of chronic pain is beyond the scope of this article, alternatives such as gabapentin, tricyclic antidepressants, and atypical antipsychotics have been used for treatment of chronic pain and can be safely prescribed during pregnancy and post partum.

A taper off of opioids can be considered during pregnancy. Although not studied in pregnancy, a dose taper of approximately 10% of the original dose every 4 to 7 days is commonly recommended and will minimize withdrawal symptoms.[33] The major concern during discontinuation of opioids during pregnancy is precipitation of physical symptoms of opioid withdrawal, mediated by increased sympathetic nervous system activity. Symptoms experienced during a slow taper are usually mild dysphoria and

---

Box 1
Checklist for patients on chronic opioid therapy during pregnancy

Checklist: care of the pregnant patient on chronic opioid therapy:

- Develop the heath care team: obstetrics, pediatrics, mental health/coping, pain medicine; any referral that can be used as an adjunct for the treatment of chronic pain (ie, physical therapy for back pain).

- Obtain release of information so all members of the team may share clinical information as needed.

- Establish who will prescribe, dose, and duration (limit to 30-day supply). If children in home, require lockbox (or equivalent) for safe storage and verify safe storage at each visit.

- Establish which provider will check the prescription monitoring system for duplicate prescriptions or medications that may increase the risk of opioid therapy (ie, sedative hypnotics, benzodiazepines).

- Establish which provider will perform urine drug screen monitoring, including frequency.

- Refer to pediatrics before delivery to discuss the neonatal plan for assessment and treatment of neonatal opioid abstinence symptoms.

- Encourage smoking cessation, as indicated.

- Develop the expectation of postpartum evaluation and treatment that will allow cessation or reduction of opioid therapy; emphasize not only personal benefit but reduced risk to children and teens in the home.

- If postpartum opioid therapy indicated, require a lockbox (or equivalent) for safe storage and verify safe storage at each visit.

anxiety. More severe symptoms of opioid withdrawal such as nausea, abdominal pain, vomiting, gooseflesh, sweating, and nasal stuffiness are uncommon with this taper. Symptoms can be managed by slowing the taper or use of ancillary medications. It would be prudent to slow or stop a taper during pregnancy if the patient experiences anything other than mild withdrawal symptoms, especially in the third trimester (24 weeks). Stewart[34] reported on detoxification from illicit opioids during pregnancy without increasing pregnancy risks (although illicit use recurred in more than 50% of women). These data should provide reassurance for the patient who would like to taper opioids prescribed for chronic pain. Concurrent care with a specialist in chronic pain can assist the obstetrician in choosing alternative plans for pain management.

Neonatal abstinence symptoms requiring treatment has been observed in 5% to 10% of neonates exposed to opioids prescribed for chronic pain; methadone exposure may increase the risk for abstinence symptoms. Pediatric consultation before delivery is recommended; delivery should take place in a care system that can evaluate and treat or refer symptomatic infants. Neonates should be closely monitored for withdrawal symptoms for 4 to 5 days after delivery.

Breastfeeding for women on chronic opioid therapy should be encouraged. Women taking codeine- or oxycodone-containing medications should be instructed how to assess the infant for lethargy and take caution when they experience medication-associated somnolence. Maternal sedation warrants special vigilance for neonatal effects and maternal dose or frequency of opioids should be reduced. Methadone is excreted at low levels in breast milk, does not require metabolism via CYP450 2D6, and could be considered for the patient prescribed regularly scheduled opioids.

In summary, risks to chronic opioid use in pregnancy for chronic pain can be reduced as follows: stop or minimize maternal smoking; stop or minimize opioid dose; consider use of alternative medications; recommend breastfeeding but parents should be aware of the symptoms of neonatal opioid intoxication; and avoid iatrogenic prematurity or early term delivery. The obstetrician should work closely with the pain specialist throughout pregnancy to discuss ancillary and alternative therapy and with the pediatrician to plan for neonatal assessment. Women who have endured chronic pain throughout a pregnancy should be encouraged to endure until at least 39 weeks to reduce neonatal morbidity.

HOW TO MINIMIZE RISK WHEN LONG-TERM OPIOID PRESCRIBING CANNOT BE AVOIDED

Chronic noncancer pain is a complex biosocial condition; the same could be said for being a new parent. Patients on chronic opioid therapy should integrate psychotherapeutic interventions, functional restoration, interdisciplinary therapy, and other adjunctive therapies for pain. These therapies should be continued during pregnancy when feasible. There are excellent clinical guidelines regarding the use of chronic opioid therapy for noncancer pain.[33,35] Any patient requiring chronic opioid therapy should be followed by a clinician with experience with chronic pain and the appropriate guidelines (**Fig. 1**).

Who should prescribe opioids during pregnancy? Ideally, the patient will have a long-standing relationship with the provider treating her chronic pain, with this relationship maintained during pregnancy. Issues such as frequency of prescriptions, assessment for desired therapeutic benefit (required for ongoing opioid therapy), and frequency of urine drug screening should occur should be outlined in the treatment plan. Most states have implemented (or have plans for) a prescription monitoring system. All prescribers of chronic opioid therapy should regularly check for

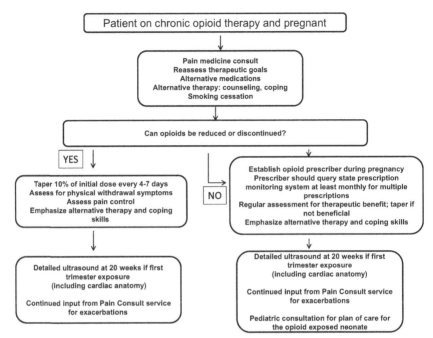

Fig. 1. Algorithm for the approach to the pregnant patient prescribed chronic opioid therapy.

prescriptions filled by a patient to avoid multiple prescriptions. This web-based system allows practitioners to see what prescriptions have been filled by a patient in that state.[36] The obstetrician should have a release of information consent to allow communication with the provider for pain medication to allow collaborative treatment.

In summary, pregnancy is an opportunity to address important issues of chronic opioid therapy in a new context. The specific benefits of smoking cessation/reduction can be reviewed. Medication storage and safety measures to reduce access to children and teens should be emphasized. Prescribing of opioids during pregnancy can be perilous, but these perils can be reduced with thoughtful conversations and patient care.

REFERENCES

1. Campbell CI, Weisner C, Leresche L, et al. Age and gender trends in long-term opioid analgesic use for noncancer pain. Am J Public Health 2010;100(12): 2541–7.
2. Kellogg A, Rose CH, Harms RH, et al. Current trends in narcotic use in pregnancy and neonatal outcomes. Am J Obstet Gynecol 2011;204:259.e1–4.
3. Darnall BD, Stacey BR, Chou R. Medical and psychological risks and consequences of long-term opioid therapy in women. Pain Med 2012;13:1181–211.
4. Lee C, Ho IK. Sex differences in opioid analgesia and addiction: interactions among opioid receptors and estrogen receptors. Pain 2013;9:45.
5. Gintzler AR, Nai-Jiang Liu NJ. Importance of sex to pain and its amelioration; relevance of spinal estrogens and its membrane receptors. Front Neuroendocrinol 2012;33:412–24.

6. Mack KA, Jones CJ, Paulozzi LJ. Vital signs: overdoses of prescription opioid pain relievers and other drugs among women- United States, 1999-2010. MMWR Morb Mortal Wkly Rep 2013;62(26):537–41.
7. Sullivan MD, Ballantyne J. What are we treating with long term opioid therapy. Arch Intern Med 2012;172(5):433–4.
8. McHugh RK, DeVito EE, Dodd D, et al. Gender differences in a clinical trial for prescription opioid dependence. J Subst Abuse Treat 2013;45:38–43.
9. Cicero TJ, Lynskey M, Todorov A, et al. Co-morbid pain and psychopathology in males and females admitted to treatment for opioid analgesic abuse. Pain 2008; 139(1):127–35.
10. Maccoun RJ. The puzzling unidimensionality of DSM-5 substance use disorder diagnoses. Front Psychiatry 2013;4:153.
11. Savage SR, Joranson DE, Covington EC, et al. Definitions related to the medical use of opioids: evolution towards universal agreement [review]. J Pain Symptom Manage 2003;26(1):655–67.
12. Bohnert AS, Valenstein M, Bair MJ, et al. Association between opioid prescribing patterns and opioid overdose-related deaths. JAMA 2011;305(13):1315–21.
13. Unick GJ, Rosenblum D, Mars S, et al. Intertwined epidemics: national demographic trends in hospitalizations for heroin- and opioid-related overdoses, 1993–2009. PLoS One 2013;8(2):e54496.
14. Hardt N, Wong T, Burt MJ, et al. Prevalence of prescription and illicit drugs inpregnancy-associated non-natural deaths of Florida mothers, 1999–2005. J Forensic Sci 2013;58(6):1536–41.
15. Burghardt LC, Ayers JW, Brownstein JS, et al. Adult prescription drug use and pediatric medication exposures and poisonings. Pediatrics 2013;132(1): 18–27.
16. McCabe SE, West BT, Boyd CJ. Leftover prescription opioids and nonmedical use among high school seniors: a multi-cohort national study. J Adolesc Health 2013;52(4):480–5.
17. Lankenau SE, Teti M, Silva K, et al. Initiation into prescription opioid misuse amongst young injection drug users. Int J Drug Policy 2012;23(1):37–44.
18. Lucke JC, Hall WD. Under what conditions is it ethical to offer incentives to encourage drug-using women to use long-acting forms of contraception? Addiction 2012;107(6):1036–41.
19. Heil SH, Jones HE, Arria A, et al. Unintended pregnancy in opioid-abusing women. J Subst Abuse Treat 2011;40(2):199–202.
20. Broussard CS, Rasmussen SA, Reefhuis J, et al, National Birth Defects Prevention Study. Maternal treatment with opioid analgesics and risk for birth defects. Am J Obstet Gynecol 2011;204(4):314.
21. You WB, Grobman W, Davis T, et al. Improving pregnancy drug warnings to promote patient comprehension. Am J Obstet Gynecol 2011;204(4):318.
22. Czeizela A, Bánhidyb F. Vitamin supply in pregnancy for prevention of congenital birth defects. Curr Opin Clin Nutr Metab Care 2011;14:291–6.
23. Bakker R, Timmermans S, Steegers EA, et al. Folic acid supplements modify the adverse effects of maternal smoking on fetal growth and neonatal complications. J Nutr 2011;141:2172–9.
24. Epstein RA, Bobo WV, Martin PR, et al. Increasing pregnancy-related use of prescribed opioid analgesics. Ann Epidemiol 2013;23(8):498–503.
25. Sharpe C, Kuschel C. Outcomes of infants born to mothers receiving methadone for pain management in pregnancy. Arch Dis Child Fetal Neonatal Ed 2004;89(1): F33–6.

26. Koren G, Cairns J, Chitayat D, et al. Pharmacogenetics of morphine poisoning in a breastfed neonate of a codeine-prescribed mother. Lancet 2006;368(9536): 704.

27. Lam J, Kelly L, Ciszkowski C, et al. Central nervous system depression of neonates breastfed by mothers receiving oxycodone for postpartum analgesia. J Pediatr 2012;160(1):33–7.

28. Juurlink DN, Gomes T, Guttmann A, et al. Postpartum maternal codeine therapy and the risk of adverse neonatal outcomes: a retrospective cohort study. Clin Toxicol (Phila) 2012;50(5):390–5.

29. NIH: Lactmed web site. Available at: http://toxnet.nlm.nih.gov/cgi-bin/sis/htmlgen? LACT. Accessed January 16, 2014.

30. Fishbain DA, Cole B, Lewis JE, et al. Is smoking associated with alcohol-drug dependence in patients with pain and chronic pain patients? An evidence-based structured review. Pain Med 2012;13(9):1212–26.

31. Jones HE, Heil SH, Tuten M, et al. Cigarette smoking in opioid-dependent pregnant women: neonatal and maternal outcomes. Drug Alcohol Depend 2013; 131(3):271–7.

32. Reeves S, Bernstein I. Effects of maternal tobacco-smoke exposure on fetal growth and neonatal size. Expert Rev Obstet Gynecol 2008;3(6):719–30.

33. Chou R, Fanciullo GJ, Fine PG, et al, American Pain Society-American Academy of Pain Medicine Opioids Guidelines Panel. Clinical guidelines for the use of chronic opioid therapy in chronic noncancer pain. J Pain 2009;10(2):113–30.

34. Stewart RD, Nelson DB, Adhikari EH, et al. The obstetrical and neonatal impact of maternal opioid detoxification in pregnancy. Am J Obstet Gynecol 2013;209(3): 267.e1–5.

35. Manchikanti L, Abdi S, Atluri S, et al. An update of comprehensive evidence-based guidelines for interventional techniques in chronic spinal pain. Part II: guidance and recommendations. Pain Physician 2013;16(Suppl 2):S49–283.

36. Reifler LM, Droz D, Bailey JE, et al. Do prescription monitoring programs impact state trends in opioid abuse/misuse? Pain Med 2012;13(3):434–42.

Fetal Surveillance in Late Pregnancy and During Labor

Luis A. Izquierdo, MD, MBA[a],*, Nicole Yonke, MD, MPH[b]

KEYWORDS

- Illegal substance abuse • Mother • Fetus • Antepartum testing

KEY POINTS

- During early gestation, drugs have teratogenic effects and can be associated with structural anomalies in the fetus.
- Substance abuse can have physiologic effects on the mother and fetus, including decreased uterine blood flow, increased vascular resistance, and an increase in fetal blood pressure.
- Women with increased risk for stillbirth should undergo antepartum fetal surveillance using a nonstress test (NST), contraction stress test, biophysical profile (BPP), or modified BPP.
- Initiating antepartum fetal testing at 32 weeks of gestation is appropriate for most pregnancies at an increased risk of stillbirth.
- Because of the high incidence of low birth weight, fetal anomalies, preterm delivery, and growth restriction, obtaining an ultrasonogram for appropriate pregnancy dating, a detailed anatomic survey, and cervical length at 20 weeks of gestation is recommended.
- In patients who are abusing stimulants such as methamphetamines and cocaine, fetal growth should be closely followed every 3 to 4 weeks and, owing to the generalized vasoconstriction that these patients develop, antenatal testing should be started routinely at 32 weeks with twice-weekly NSTs and a once-weekly modified BPP.

INTRODUCTION

Once gestation is beyond 20 weeks, clinicians have to address the impact of illicit substances on fetal growth, placentation, and the possibility of early delivery. Cannabis remains the most commonly used illicit drug in the United States.[1] Other agents used by pregnant patients include heroin, cocaine, hallucinogens, inhalants, alcohol,

The authors have nothing to disclose.
[a] Division of Maternal Fetal Medicine, University of New Mexico School of Medicine, MSC 105580, 1 University of New Mexico, Albuquerque, NM 87131, USA; [b] Division of Maternal Child Health, University of New Mexico School of Medicine, 1 University of New Mexico, Albuquerque, NM 87131, USA
* Corresponding author.
E-mail address: lizquierdo@salud.unm.edu

Obstet Gynecol Clin N Am 41 (2014) 307–315
http://dx.doi.org/10.1016/j.ogc.2014.02.009
0889-8545/14/$ – see front matter © 2014 Elsevier Inc. All rights reserved.

and prescription psychotherapeutics.[2] An estimated 4.4% of pregnant women report illicit drug use in the preceding 30 days.[3] During early gestation drugs have teratogenic effects, and can be associated with structural anomalies in the fetus.[4,5] Substance abuse can have physiologic effects on the mother and fetus, including decreased uterine blood flow, increased vascular resistance, and an increase in fetal blood pressure.[1] As pregnancy advances, these substances can have more subtle effects that can lead to abnormal fetal growth, alterations in fetal growth, alterations in neurotransmitters and their receptors, and brain organization.

The effects of illegal substance abuse during pregnancy should be addressed with caution given the nature of the available evidence. Investigators have raised at least 4 issues that are of particular concern when analyzing these data:

1. The difficulty of accurately measuring illicit substance-use patterns in women throughout pregnancy.
2. The difficulty in separating the effects of drug use from the effects of other adverse confounding personal and social circumstances.
3. The existence of a common pattern of polysubstance use in this population.
4. Possible publication bias or apparent reviewer editorial bias that results in preferential publication in the scientific literature of studies that show unfavorable outcomes in association with substance use.[6]

This article describes the effects of substance use during pregnancy on fetal growth and surveillance in the antepartum and intrapartum period, based on the research available and the authors' own clinical experience.

MATERNAL AND FETAL CONSEQUENCES OF ILLICIT SUBSTANCE USE IN PREGNANCY
Marijuana or Cannabis

As already mentioned, marijuana is one of the most commonly used drugs in the United States during pregnancy, and its use appears to be increasing steadily in those aged 12 years or older.[3] Δ9-Tetrahydrocannabinol is the active ingredient in marijuana, and readily crosses the placenta. Of importance is that marijuana produces higher blood carboxyhemoglobin levels than are produced by cigarette smoking. These higher concentrations of carboxyhemoglobin can affect fetal oxygenation and, ultimately, fetal growth and development.[3]

Opioids

Addiction to opioids can develop by repetitive use of either prescription opioid analgesics or heroin.[4] Heroin is a highly addictive substance with a short half-life, which can be injected, smoked, or nasally inhaled. Commonly prescribed opioids such as codeine, fentanyl, morphine, methadone, oxycodone, and hydrocodone are the most burgeoning drugs of abuse in the United States.[4,7] Although the usual route of administration of these medications is oral, they are also injected, nasally inhaled, smoked, used as dermal patches, or used as suppositories.[4] All of these agents have the potential for overdose, abuse, addiction, and physical dependence.

The continued use of illicit opioids and the associated lifestyle represents the greatest threat to the well-being of the mother, fetus, and neonate.[8] Severe opioid withdrawal can lead to fetal death because of the offspring's experience of acute opioid abstinence syndrome.[4] Untreated heroin use is associated with an increased risk of fetal growth restriction, abruptio placenta, fetal death, preterm labor, and intrauterine passage of meconium.[3] Compared with nonusers, heroin abuse increases the risk of a mother having a low birth weight neonate 4.6-fold.[3]

Infants exposed to opioids in utero also are at risk of developing neonatal abstinence syndrome (NAS). NAS is categorized by increased central nervous system excitability, and in many cases results in the need for pharmacologic withdrawal treatment.[8] Methadone and buprenorphine can be used to treat opioid cravings and withdrawals to help women abstain from using heroin. Although methadone has traditionally been the standard of care, newer data demonstrate the safety of buprenorphine use during pregnancy. The risk of NAS and hospitalization stay after birth is lower for infants exposed to buprenorphine than to methadone.[9,10] Buprenorphine has also been associated with higher birth weight in comparison with methadone.[10] The data comparing infants exposed to methadone with unexposed infants is mixed, with some studies demonstrating an increased risk of low birth weight and others demonstrating no difference.[3,11]

Cocaine

Cocaine blocks the presynaptic reuptake of the sympathomimetic neurotransmitters such as norepinephrine, serotonin, and dopamine, resulting in hypertension, tachycardia, and even cardiac arrhythmias.[12] Because of its sympathomimetic vasoconstrictive effects and resultant hypertension in both the mother and the fetus, placental infarcts and hemorrhage can occur at any time during pregnancy.[6] Cocaine exposure during pregnancy directly alters the uteroplacental blood flow, resulting in fetal and neonatal sequelae. Cocaine crosses the placental barrier easily, with amniotic fluid acting as a reservoir for fetal cocaine exposure. The overall malformation rate in pregnancies exposed to cocaine is around 10%.[4] Perinatal cocaine use has been associated with preterm birth, low birth weight, and small for gestational age (SGA) infants.[6] Nonetheless, some of the perinatal adverse effects commonly attributed to cocaine may be caused by confounders associated with its use.[13]

No pharmacologic substitutes have been identified for the effective treatment of stimulant abuse. The Cochrane Database reviews have evaluated antidepressants, anticonvulsants, and dopamine agonist agents for cocaine dependence, and have not shown benefit to derive from any such therapies.[14]

Amphetamines

In the United States it is estimated that 5% of pregnant women have used methamphetamines.[1] In animal models, methamphetamines have been found to decrease uterine blood flow, increase uterine vascular resistance, and increase fetal blood pressure in dose-related fashion.[1] Amphetamine and its derivatives, methamphetamine and methylenedioxymethamphetamine (MDMA), are slowly metabolized and easily distributed to the central nervous system. Of note, amphetamine derivatives have longer half-lives and have more sympathomimetic properties than cocaine. After exposure to amphetamines, the elevated levels of circulating neurotransmitters (norepinephrine and serotonin) produce marked vasoconstriction and lead to adverse perinatal effects.[1] Amphetamine exposure in pregnancy is associated with higher unadjusted odds of preterm birth, low birth weight, and SGA neonates.[1]

Alcohol

Prenatal alcohol exposure has been reported by 12.5% of pregnant women, with 1.6% reporting frequent use of alcohol while pregnant.[15] Binge drinking ($\geq$4 drinks per occasion) has been estimated at 1.4% among pregnant women and 15% among nonpregnant women in the United States during the period 2006 to 2010. Factors related to maternal alcohol consumption during pregnancy and preconception binge drinking include maternal age, whether the pregnancy was planned, abuse of other substances, marital status, history of physical and emotional abuse, mental health, self-esteem, prenatal care, nutrition, and socioeconomic status.[16] Regarding morbidity and mortality related to alcohol exposure, excessive alcohol consumption is the third leading preventable cause of death in the United States, and is estimated to be responsible for approximately 80,000 deaths annually. Alcohol can be a significant contributing factor to medical conditions such as hepatitis, hypertension, tuberculosis, pneumonia, pancreatitis, and cardiomyopathy.[17] Fifty percent of all cases of cirrhosis in the United States have been found to be due to alcohol-use disorders. Excessive alcohol consumption also contributes to cancers of the mouth, esophagus, pharynx, larynx, and breast. Alcohol abuse inflicts central nervous system disease including dementia, stroke, and peripheral nervous system disease such as neuropathy and myopathy.[18]

Prenatal alcohol exposure has been found to be a risk factor for fetal mortality, stillbirth, and infant and child mortality. One or 2 hours after maternal ingestion, the fetal blood alcohol concentrations reach levels nearly equivalent to maternal levels.[15] Fetal exposure time is prolonged, arising from reuptake by the fetus of the amniotic fluid containing ethanol. Fetal alcohol exposure increases the risk of extreme preterm delivery.[19] Research has also found that alcohol consumption during pregnancy increases the risk of fetal death.

ANTEPARTUM FETAL EVALUATION OF WOMEN USING ILLICIT DRUGS

The goal of antepartum fetal evaluation is to decrease perinatal mortality and permanent neurologic injury through judicious use of reliable and valid methods of fetal assessment (**Fig. 1**).[20,21]

Women with increased risk for stillbirth should undergo antepartum fetal surveillance using a nonstress test (NST), contraction stress test (CST), biophysical profile (BPP), or modified BPP. Initiating this testing at 32 weeks of gestation is appropriate

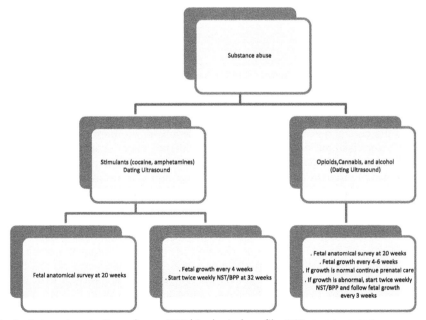

Fig. 1. Antepartum testing scheme. BPP, biophysical profile; NST, nonstress test.

for most pregnancies at an increased risk of stillbirth.[21] In all these testing schemes, the prevalence of the abnormal condition will have a great impact on the predictive value of the antenatal tests and the number needed to evaluate with testing and to treat with interventions; that is, delivery to presumably prevent fetal death.[20]

Several tests are available to engage in close surveillance of patients at risk. Fetal movements or kick counts is a more indirect indicator of fetal oxygenation, because decreased fetal movements occur in response to hypoxemia. Studies performed to assess fetal movement counts have failed to conclusively show benefits in the prevention of perinatal mortality.[20,21] The NST is based on the premise that the heart rate of the fetus that is not acidotic or neurologically depressed will temporarily accelerate with fetal movement.[21] Fetal heart rate reactivity is thought to be a good indicator of normal fetal autonomic function, whereas loss or reactivity is associated most commonly with a fetal sleep cycle, but it may result from any cause of central nervous system depression including fetal acidosis.[20,21]

The CST, or oxytocin challenge test, is based on the fact the uterine contractions produce reductions in the blood flow in the intervillous space. An inadequate placenta respiratory reserve would demonstrate recurrent late decelerations in response to hypoxia.[20,21]

The BPP consists of an NST combined with 4 observations made by real-time ultrasonography. The 5 components are the NST, the fetal breathing movements, the fetal movements, the fetal tone, and the determination of the amniotic fluid volume.[21] The BPP correlates well with a fetal acid-base status. A modified BPP is based on the fact that the amniotic fluid reflects fetal urine production. If there is placental dysfunction, this may result in diminished fetal renal profusion, leading to oligohydramnios. Amniotic fluid volume can therefore be used to evaluate long-term uteroplacental dysfunction. As discussed earlier, the NST is a short-term indicator of the fetal acid-base status when combined with the amniotic fluid index (AFI), which is the sum of measurements of the deepest cord-free amniotic fluid pocket in each abdominal quadrant; these 2 tests serve as an indicator of long-term placental function.[21]

It is also important to mention the use of ultrasonography in women involved with substance abuse. Ultrasonography can be used to diagnose many major fetal anomalies. Prenatal ultrasonography may reduce the rate of perinatal mortality, primarily through pregnancy termination for prenatal diagnosed congenital anomalies, but does not appear to reduce the rate of perinatal morbidity. Ultrasonography also provides a more accurate estimation of gestational age, which prevents unnecessary labor induction for postterm pregnancy.[22] Ultrasonographic examination between 18 and 20 weeks of gestation allows for a reasonable survey of fetal anatomy and an accurate estimation of gestational age. Therefore, the optimal timing for a single ultrasonogram is between 18 and 20 weeks, because anatomically complex organs such as the fetal heart and brain can be imaged with sufficient clarity to allow detection of many major malformations at a time when termination of pregnancy may still be an option. Other uses of ultrasonography during pregnancy are the evaluation of cervical length, determination of gestational age, evaluation of amniotic fluid, detection of disturbances of fetal growth, and detection of chromosomal abnormalities in the second trimester.[22]

ANTEPARTUM TESTING GUIDELINES FOR PATIENTS WITH SUBSTANCE ABUSE

Because of the high incidence of low birth weight, fetal anomalies, preterm delivery, and growth restriction, the authors recommend obtaining an ultrasonogram for appropriate pregnancy dating, a detailed anatomic survey, and cervical length at 20 weeks of gestation. The authors also perform urine drug screens during every clinic visit to assess whether these patients are using or abusing other substances.

Pregnant women with active substance abuse can be cared for in specialized prenatal clinics designed to care for women with addiction, or by individual prenatal providers with experience in addiction medicine. At the time women establish care, an initial ultrasonogram for assessment of gestational age is recommended. These patients may also be offered the opportunity for aneuploidy screening in the first and second trimester. An anatomic survey of the fetus is obtained at 20 weeks. The progress of the pregnancy is assessed by frequent prenatal visits and fundal height.

If there is sufficient discrepancy in the growth to suspect macrosomia or growth restriction, ultrasonography is repeated. Women in the authors' specialized substance-abuse prenatal clinic have a higher incidence of intrauterine growth restriction in comparison with other women delivering at the institution. Although it is unclear whether this finding is due to active substance abuse, opioid substitution therapy, or confounders such as tobacco abuse and poor weight gain, growth ultrasonograms on women at 28 and 34 weeks' gestation are routinely obtained to screen for intrauterine growth restriction. The authors do not routinely perform antenatal testing in this population. If a fetal growth disorder is identified, the mother is followed with twice-weekly NSTs starting at 32 weeks, and weekly AFIs or modified BPPs.

In patients who are abusing stimulants such as methamphetamines and cocaine, fetal growth is followed every 3 to 4 weeks. Because of the generalized vasoconstriction that these patients develop, antenatal testing is started routinely at 32 weeks with twice-weekly NSTs and a once-weekly modified BPP. Also of importance is that opioid substitution therapy affects fetal assessment by NST and BPP. A decrease in fetal heart rate can be found in opioid-dependent mothers as early as the first trimester.[23] After methadone administration, the reactivity of NSTs decreases.[24] The baseline heart rate is also slower, with fewer accelerations and decreased variability.[8] Buprenorphine, compared with methadone, is less likely to have these effects.[25]

Intrapartum Management

In women with active stimulant abuse, the authors routinely induce labor at 38 weeks of gestation because of the increased risk of abruptio placenta, balancing this risk with the risk of prematurity. Owing to this higher incidence of abruptio placenta secondary to cocaine and methamphetamine abuse, it is recommended that women using stimulants be placed on continuous fetal monitoring and be observed for hypertonic contractions. The limited use of short-acting benzodiazepines is allowed for symptomatic relief of severe agitation from stimulant withdrawal, if needed, during inpatient care.[9,14,26]

As with antepartum interpretation of NSTs, methadone also affects intrapartum fetal heart rate patterns, with a decreased fetal heart rate baseline, fewer accelerations, and decreased variability.[27–30] Women receiving opioid substitution therapy undergoing labor should receive routine pain relief as if they were not taking opioids, because the maintenance dose does not provide adequate analgesia for labor.[4] Epidural or spinal anesthesia should be offered, where appropriate, for management of pain in labor or for delivery. Narcotic agonist-antagonist drugs such as butorphanol and nalbuphine should be avoided because they may precipitate an acute opioid withdrawal.[4] As a general rule, patients undergoing opioid maintenance treatment will require higher dosages of opioids to achieve an analgesic effect in comparison with other patients.[4] The authors do not stop buprenorphine therapy in labor or for cesarean sections. Instead, the dose of buprenorphine is divided 3 to 4 times throughout the day to improve its analgesic effect, and the dose of the other opioids given for pain control is increased.

SUMMARY

This article addresses the effects of illegal and legal substance abuse on both mother and fetus, and discusses the antepartum and intrapartum management of substance-abusing patients. When assessing the impact of illicit drug exposure on pregnancy, clinicians are confronted with several common confounders, including tobacco use, limited use of and access to prenatal care, polysubstance exposure, lack of insurance coverage, low socioeconomic status, and improper nutrition.[1] The evidence presented suggests that exposure to substance abuse during pregnancy has a negative effect on the birth weight, gestational age at delivery, fetal growth, and the possibility of abruptio placenta. Once identified, these patients should ideally attend a specialized clinic where comprehensive care of perinatal substance abuse can be provided. These specialized clinics can improve maternal and perinatal outcomes. Not only is the fetus placed at risk in these situations but the mother is also at risk for hypertensive disorders, cardiovascular fluctuations, and placental abruption, as well as maternal mortality in some situations.

There is evidence that perinatal outcomes improve in some of the monitored populations who undergo fetal assessment.[7] The American College of Obstetricians and Gynecologists suggest starting fetal monitoring at between 32 and 34 weeks. However, fetal testing should be individualized according to which high-risk disorder affects the fetus.[7,21] At the authors' institution, antepartum testing protocols for the substance abuse population are started at 32 weeks of gestation. In those cases presenting with evidence of growth restriction before 32 weeks it is recommended that testing protocols should begin earlier, around 28 weeks' gestation.

Antepartum complications, such as substance abuse, can lead to uteroplacental insufficiency and intrapartum events that can result in adverse neonatal outcomes. The labor of women with such high-risk conditions should be monitored with continuous fetal heart rate monitoring. In these circumstances a 3-tiered system for the categorizations of fetal heart rate patterns is recommended.[11]

In essence, clinicians need to make their best effort to identify patients with substance addictions and thus be able to provide adequate maternal and fetal care.

REFERENCES

1. Ladhani NN, Shah PS, Murphy KE. Prenatal amphetamine exposure and birth outcomes: a systematic review and metaanalysis. Am J Obstet Gynecol 2011; 205:219.e1–7.
2. Varner MW, Silver RM, Rowland-Hogue CJ, et al. Association between stillbirth and illicit drug use and smoking during pregnancy. Obstet Gynecol 2014;123: 113–25.
3. Soto E, Bahado-Singh R. Fetal abnormal growth associated with substance abuse. Clin Obstet Gynecol 2013;56(1):142–53.
4. American College of Obstetricians and Gynecologists. Opioid abuse, dependence, and addiction in pregnancy. Committee Opinion No. 524. Obstet Gynecol 2012;119:1070–6.
5. Behnke M, Smith VC. Prenatal substance abuse: short and long term outcome on the exposed fetus. Pediatrics 2013;131:e1009–25.
6. Gouin K, Murphy K, Shah P. Effects of cocaine use during pregnancy on low birth weight and preterm birth: systematic review and metaanalysis. Am J Obstet Gynecol 2011;204:340.e1–12.
7. Creasy RK, Resnik R, Iams JD, et al. Creasy and Rensik's maternal fetal medicine, principles and practice. Philadelphia: Elsevier Saunders; 2014.

8. Kakko J, Heilig M, Sarman I. Buprenorphine and methadone treatment of opiate dependence during pregnancy: comparison of fetal growth and neonatal outcome in two consecutive case series. Drug Alcohol Depend 2008;96:69–78.

9. Center for Substance Abuse Treatment. Medication assisted treatment for opioid addiction in opioid treatment programs (Treatment Improvement Protocol Series 43). Rockville (MD): US Department of Health and Human Services; 2005.

10. Centers for Disease Control and Prevention. CDC grand rounds: prescription drug overdoses—a U.S. epidemic. MMWR Morb Mortal Wkly Rep 2012;61:10–3.

11. American College of Obstetricians and Gynecologists. Intrapartum fetal heart rate monitoring: nomenclature, interpretation and general management principles. ACOG Practice Bulletin 106. Obstet Gynecol 2009;114:192–202.

12. Cain MA, Bornick P, Whiteman V. The maternal, fetal, and neonatal effects on cocaine exposure in pregnancy. Clin Obstet Gynecol 2013;56(1):124–32.

13. Addis A, Moretti MY, Syed FA, et al. Fetal effects of cocaine: an updated metaanalysis. Reprod Toxicol 2001;15:341–69.

14. Srisurapanont M, Jarusuraisin N, Kittirattanappaiboon P. Treatment of amphetamine dependence and abuse. Cochrane Database Syst Rev 2008;(4): CD006754.

15. Burd L, Blair J, Dropps K. Prenatal alcohol exposure, blood alcohol concentrations, and alcohol elimination rates for the mother, fetus and newborn. J Perinatol 2012;32:652–9.

16. Zelner I, Koren G. Alcohol consumption among women. J Popul Ther Clin Pharmacol 2013;20:e201–6.

17. Zaridze D, Brennan P, Boreham J, et al. Alcohol and cause-specific mortality in Russia: a retrospective case-control study of 48557 adult deaths. Lancet 2009; 373:2201–14.

18. Thun MJ, Peto R, Lopez AD, et al. Alcohol consumption and mortality among middle aged and elderly US adults. N Engl J Med 1997;337:1705–14.

19. Jones TB, Bailey BA, Sokol RJ. Alcohol use in pregnancy: insights in screening and intervention for the clinician. Clin Obstet Gynecol 2013;56(1):114–23.

20. Gabbe SG, Niebyl JE, Simpson JL, et al, editors. Obstetrics normal and problem pregnancies. Philadelphia: Elsevier Saunders; 2012.

21. American College of Obstetricians and Gynecologists Recommendations. Anterpartum fetal surveillance. Practice bulletin 9. October 1999. Reaffirmed 2012.

22. American College of Obstetricians and Gynecologists Recommendations. Ultrasonography in pregnancy. Practice bulletin number 101. February 2009. Reaffirmed 2012.

23. Cleary BJ, Eogan M, O'Connell MP, et al. Methadone and perinatal outcomes: a prospective cohort study. Addiction 2012;107:1482–92.

24. Jones HE, Kaltenbach K, Heil SH, et al. Neonatal abstinence syndrome after methadone or buprenorphine exposure. N Engl J Med 2010;363:2320–31.

25. Schmid M, Kuessel L, Klein K, et al. First-trimester fetal heart rate in mothers with opioid addiction. Addiction 2010;105:1265–8.

26. Medscape. Illicit drug use in pregnancy: effects and management: labor, delivery, and breast feeding. New York: Medscape; 2011. Available at: http://www. medscape.org/vienarticle/738688_10. Accessed January 20, 2014.

27. Archie CL, Lee MI, Sokol RJ, et al. The effects of methadone treatment on the reactivity of the nonstress test. Obstet Gynecol 1989;74:254–5.

28. Jansson LM, Dipietro J, Elko A. Fetal response to maternal methadone administration. Am J Obstet Gynecol 2005;193:611–7.

29. Salisbury AL, Coyle MG, O'Grady KE, et al. Fetal assessment before and after dosing with buprenorphine or methadone. Addiction 2012;107(Suppl 1):36–44.
30. Ramirez-Cacho WA, Flores S, Schrader RM, et al. Effect of chronic maternal methadone therapy on intrapartum fetal heart rate patterns. J Soc Gynecol Investig 2006;13:108–11.

Neonatal Opioid Withdrawal Syndrome

Mary Beth Sutter, MD[a], Lawrence Leeman, MD, MPH[b],*, Andrew Hsi, MD[c]

KEYWORDS

- Neonatal abstinence syndrome • Neonatal opioid withdrawal
- Perinatal substance abuse • Buprenorphine • Methadone

KEY POINTS

- It is important for all providers to recognize neonatal opioid withdrawal with shifts in maternal prescription opioid use and abuse.
- Current evidence points to a milder withdrawal syndrome with maternal buprenorphine maintenance in comparison with methadone.
- Initial treatment of neonatal opioid withdrawal should be with opioid monotherapy; currently there is no evidence to recommend one regimen over another. Adjunctive therapy, if required, should be with phenobarbital or clonidine.
- The hospital environment should be maximized to promote low stimuli for infants affected by withdrawal, and should include rooming-in and breastfeeding promotion where appropriate.
- At present there is limited evidence on the long-term childhood effects of perinatal opioid exposure, and support is needed for families during early childhood development.

BACKGROUND AND EPIDEMIOLOGY

Neonates who have had in utero exposures from maternal substance abuse can experience central nervous system effects of the drugs, including drug toxicity and withdrawal. Neonatal abstinence syndrome (NAS), initially described in the 1970s, is the term used for the constellation of withdrawal symptoms. The clinical features and treatment of withdrawal from opioids is a specific form of NAS, and has recently been termed neonatal opioid withdrawal syndrome (NOWS). This review focuses primarily on the presentation, diagnosis, and management of NOWS, with emphasis on current evidence for assessment by scoring systems, pharmacologic treatment protocols, and implications for future policy and research.

The authors have nothing to disclose.

[a] Department of Family and Community Medicine, University of New Mexico, 2400 Tucker North East, MSC09 5040, Albuquerque, NM 87131, USA; [b] Departments of Family and Community Medicine, Obstetrics & Gynecology, University of New Mexico, 2400 Tucker North East, MSC09 5040, NM 87131, USA; [c] Department of Pediatrics, University of New Mexico, MSC10 5590, Albuquerque, NM, USA
* Corresponding author.
E-mail address: lleeman@salud.unm.edu

The rising incidence of maternal opioid use is demonstrated by hospital discharge records revealing a nationwide increase from 1.19 to 5.63 per 1000 births per year from 2000 to 2009.[1] In 2012, an estimated 5.9% of women aged 15 to 44 years were using illicit drugs during pregnancy.[2] Marijuana use is most common, followed by use of prescription opioids and, less commonly, stimulants, heroin, and psychotropic drugs.[3] Unique to the past several years is the rapid increase in prescription opioid abuse,[1,4] which has changed both the number and demographic characteristics of pregnant women using illicit substances, necessitating providers of all geographic and socioeconomic populations to be aware of the management of neonatal opioid withdrawal.

The epidemic abuse of prescription opioids and continued heroin use have increased the rates of NAS from 1.20 per 1000 births in 2000 to 3.39 per 1000 births in 2009, with an estimated 1 newborn per hour born with NAS in the United States in 2009.[1] Health care spending for illicit drug use during pregnancy and related neonatal outcomes has increased from an average of US$39,400 per NAS hospital admission in 2000 to $53,400 in 2009, with 77.6% of these charges attributed to state Medicaid in 2009.[1] The length of stay for NAS averages 16 days and has not significantly changed during this time.[1] According to a recent survey, only about half of neonatal intensive care units (NICUs) in the United States have a written protocol for the diagnosis and management of NAS, which represents an important area for educational improvement.[5]

CLINICAL PRESENTATION AND DIAGNOSIS

Mothers who are abusing opioids may be identified during prenatal care and referred to perinatal substance abuse programs, which will optimally have an affiliated neonatal program. Unfortunately many women with opioid addiction do not obtain prenatal care, and are first seen when they present in labor. Some women, particularly those with addiction to prescription opioids, may be able to obtain a prescription from other physicians or purchase diverted "street drugs" during the pregnancy, and the neonatal exposure will be unsuspected until the withdrawal syndrome develops. Risk factors for maternal drug abuse include poor or no prenatal care, a previously unexplained late fetal demise placental abruption, unexplained intrauterine growth restriction, maternal hypertension, and precipitous labor.[6,7] These factors, clinical suspicion of opioid withdrawal, or a known history of maternal drug abuse or opioid replacement therapy may prompt screening with a maternal or neonatal urine drug screen or meconium toxicology testing. The legal implications of this screening are important to consider before initiation, as several states consider a positive newborn urine drug screen to be evidence of child abuse.[8] The optimal urine sample for neonatal screening is the first urine after birth, as many substances are quickly metabolized and become undetectable.[7] Urine testing can result in false positives, as some prescription medications and over-the-counter products cross-react with testing for drugs of abuse, so that a positive test on the screening procedure requires confirmatory testing by gas chromatography or mass spectrometry.[8] Drugs that are metabolized by the fetal liver and kidneys are concentrated in meconium, which can detect prenatal substance exposure that has occurred months before birth; therefore, meconium testing may be positive when urine testing is negative.[7,8] Analysis of neonatal hair or umbilical cord tissue can also provide a window of screening of weeks to months, but are primarily used only for research purposes at present.[8]

The probability of newborns exposed to maternal chronic opioid use developing withdrawal symptoms that are sufficient to require pharmacologic therapy varies widely in studies, and likely depends on the composite of substances prescribed to or abused by the mother as well as genetic, epigenetic, and environmental factors.[9] The effects of illicit drugs on fetal development are related primarily to abnormal growth and alterations in neurotransmitters and brain development, rather than major structural teratogenic effects.[10] Beyond the drugs themselves, behaviors of women who chronically abuse substances may also lead to neonatal problems resulting from poor access to or compliance with prenatal care, poor nutrition resulting in reduced delivery of nutrients to the fetus, increased rates of mental illness and interpersonal violence, and exposure to infections including human immunodeficiency virus (HIV) and hepatitis C.[9,11]

Opioid exposure in utero leads to a well-described complex of withdrawal signs and symptoms that can be described as NOWS. Studies have shown that 21% to 94% of neonates exposed to opioids in utero will develop withdrawal signs and symptoms that are severe enough to warrant pharmacologic treatment.[7,12,13] Factors that affect the likelihood and severity of NOWS include the specific opioid exposure, dose of opioid replacement therapy, gestational age, polysubstance abuse, tobacco, and breastfeeding.

Methadone, a full opioid μ-receptor agonist, has been the standard of care for opioid treatment in pregnancy in the United States since the 1970s.[14] The use of buprenorphine, a partial μ-receptor antagonist, for opioid addiction in pregnancy appears to have increased rapidly since the 2010 MOTHER trial, and other recent studies, demonstrated less severe neonatal opioid withdrawal and equivalent obstetric outcomes.[9,15–17] Several studies have demonstrated that the dose of methadone replacement therapy is not related to the incidence or severity of withdrawal, and methadone should be titrated to alleviate maternal withdrawal symptoms and cravings for illicit drug use.[18–21] However, other studies have shown a higher likelihood of infants requiring pharmacologic treatment for withdrawal with higher doses of methadone, especially when increased or initiated near term, or when combined with benzodiazepine abuse.[22–26] Women who have been on long-term methadone maintenance therapy before conception appear to have more favorable outcomes.[27] Most experts agree that maternal methadone treatment should not be decreased to prevent neonatal withdrawal severity, as the higher likelihood of a relapse of opioid abuse increases the incidence of poor pregnancy outcomes, including intrauterine growth restriction and preterm delivery.[28,29] Compared with methadone-exposed infants, buprenorphine-exposed infants in the MOTHER trial required less morphine, had shorter hospital stays, and had a shorter duration of treatment for neonatal withdrawal syndrome, with no significant differences in adverse maternal or neonatal outcomes.[17] There is also no evidence for a dose-response relationship between maternal buprenorphine dose at the time of delivery and neonatal outcomes, including severity of withdrawal or need for pharmacologic treatment.[30] In one study, male infants exposed to buprenorphine had higher mean withdrawal scores and required pharmacologic therapy more often than their female counterparts, possibly pointing to a gender-specific association.[31] This same relationship has been disproved with methadone-exposed infants.[32] Differences in neonatal withdrawal with methadone and buprenorphine are described in **Box 1**.

Symptoms of NOWS commonly begin within 24 to 72 hours after birth, the average time of onset being dependent on the half-life of the substance. The American Academy of Pediatrics recommends observation of opioid-exposed neonates in the hospital for 3 days for short-acting opioids and up to 5 to 7 days for long-acting opioids,[7] as the need for initiation of pharmacologic treatment can occur up to 120 hours of life.[6,7,9] Infants exposed to minimal episodic use of opioids for medical indications such as

---

Box 1
Methadone versus buprenorphine in neonatal withdrawal

Methadone	Buprenorphine
Full μ-receptor agonist	Partial μ-receptor antagonist
Likely no dose-response relationship[18]	No dose-response relationship[30]
Likely no gender-specific relationship[32]	
Possible faster time to withdrawal[34]	Possible slower time to withdrawal[34]
Increased severity with benzodiazepenes[39]	Lower peak Finnegan scores[17]
	Shorter hospital stays[17]
	Shorter duration of treatment[17]

---

migraine headache or musculoskeletal pain appear to be at minimal risk for neonatal withdrawal requiring pharmacologic treatment; however, it is often difficult to assess the degree of exposure. When the degree of exposure is uncertain, the authors recommend observing infants in the hospital for at least 96 hours. Studies of methadone concentration in cord blood have noted that lower starting concentrations of methadone and more rapid decline in levels are associated with more severe symptoms of withdrawal.[33] In one study, infants exposed to methadone in utero had a shorter time to withdrawal than infants exposed to buprenorphine, independent of other demographic factors (34 vs 71 hours).[34] The pathophysiology of neonatal opioid withdrawal can be explained by the presence of opioid receptors in the brain and gastrointestinal tract, leading to mostly central nervous system, autonomic system, and gastrointestinal signs and symptoms.[7] Signs and symptoms are summarized in **Box 2**.

Several features of opioid withdrawal in neonates are nonspecific and may be associated with other serious conditions. The knowledge of maternal substance abuse during pregnancy should not preclude careful consideration of a differential diagnosis, including infection, hypoglycemia, hypocalcemia, hyperthyroidism, intracranial hemorrhage, hypoxic-ischemic encephalopathy, or maternal use of selective serotonin reuptake inhibitors (SSRIs).[7]

Several special populations may present differently from the classic syndrome described. Preterm infants may have less severe or less prolonged presentations because of neurologic immaturity, less cumulative drug exposure, or less drug retained in fat stores.[7,26] Infants affected by maternal polysubstance abuse may have differing presentations from those exposed to opioids alone.[35] Benzodiazepines, though not well studied, can cause a withdrawal picture similar to opioid withdrawal including hypertonia, hyperreflexia, tremors, vomiting, hyperactivity, and tachypnea.[7,36] Withdrawal from benzodiazepines can therefore cloud the clinical picture and potentially lead to prolonged treatment of opioid withdrawal.[35,36] SSRIs also have a similar withdrawal picture in neonates, including irritability, poor suck, feeding difficulties, tremors, hypertonia, tachypnea, and sleep disturbances, although symptoms are usually not severe enough to require medication.[7,37,38] In a 2008 study from Boston, benzodiazepine use combined with methadone use significantly increased the length of stay in hospital by 5.88 days in comparison with methadone alone.[39] This finding was similar to those of prior studies of concurrent methadone and benzodiazepine use, which also showed an increased length of neonatal hospitalization for withdrawal.[24,25] In these same studies, neither maternal SSRI use nor tobacco use while on methadone increased adverse outcomes.[25,39] However, other studies have shown higher peak NAS scores among infants born to women smoking 20 or more cigarettes a day when compared with lighter or never smokers.[40]

Box 2
Clinical features of neonatal opioid withdrawal

Central Nervous System

  High-pitched cry

  Irritability

  Exaggerated primitive reflexes

  Hyperactive deep tendon reflexes

  Increased tone

  Altered sleep-wake cycles

  Tremors

  Seizures

Gastrointestinal

  Vomiting

  Loose stools

  Poor feeding

  Uncoordinated, constant sucking

  Failure to thrive

Autonomic Dysfunction

  Sweating

  Sneezing

  Temperature instability

  Nasal stuffiness

  Yawning

Adapted from Hudak ML, Tan RC, Committee on Drugs, Committee on Fetus and Newborn, American Academy of Pediatrics. Neonatal drug withdrawal. Pediatrics 2012;129:e540–60.

PATHOPHYSIOLOGY OF NEONATAL OPIOID WITHDRAWAL

The pathophysiology of neonatal opioid withdrawal includes the contributions of fetal genetics, fetal response to maternal withdrawal symptoms stemming from reduced levels of opioids passed to fetal circulation, effects of stress responses in the fetus in reaction to maternal physical condition, and evidence of abnormalities in brain electrical activity as observed by continuous electroencephalographic (EEG) monitoring. The fetal propensity for neonatal opioid withdrawal may be influenced by the genes responsible for 2 proteins associated with opioid addiction in adults. The single-nucleotide polymorphisms affecting the μ-opioid receptor (*OPRM1*) and catechol-*O* methyltransferase (*COMT*) genes have an association with greater risk of adult addiction to opioids.[41] These polymorphisms have protective effects for infants treated for neonatal opioid withdrawal, including shortened length of hospital stay, less need for any pharmacologic treatment, and less need for treatment with 2 or more medications.[41]

    The likelihood of an infant developing opioid withdrawal may be associated with the timing and quantity of opioids transferred to the developing fetal brain. The duration of use of a specific dose of any opioid that is sufficient to result in neonatal withdrawal is unknown and, as previously described, the literature has contradictory findings regarding the effects of methadone dose on neonatal risk of withdrawal.[18,23,24] The variability of purity of street heroin in communities over time combined with the intermittent availability of opioids being procured for substance abuse may result in intrauterine fetal withdrawal. Neither disclosure of extent and duration of opioid use, nor current methods of detection of opioids in biological fluids, can accurately estimate the extent of exposure to the fetus.

The clinical features of neonatal opioid withdrawal include observed seizures, which are often more heavily weighted in the scoring system, suggesting a relationship to more severe withdrawal. Clinical observation may not detect subtler abnormalities of electrical transmission in the brain as evidenced by continuous amplitude-integrated EEG tracings, as one study found that 6 of 8 infants exposed to opioids had subclinical seizures that did not require treatment in the first 3 days of life.[42]

Sleep disorganization contributes to the severity of opioid withdrawal, as shown by continuous EEG monitoring of patients receiving treatment for NAS compared with nonopioid-exposed controls.[43] The observations of disordered sleep accompanied by subclinical seizures suggest alterations of brain electrical activity, which may correlate with clinical observations of a delay in opioid-exposed infants developing normal sleep-wake cycles in the first months of life.

Conceptualization of the pathophysiology of neonatal opioid withdrawal may in the future include genetic analysis to guide interventions; however, clinicians will continue to apply clinical expertise to guide such interventions. The brain disturbances revealed by continuous EEG monitoring may provide greater fine-tuning for intervention during hospitalization. The maturation of brain systems and the effects on the clinical scoring as infants mature may result in a need to adjust clinical evaluation and NAS scoring for those infants hospitalized for longer stays. An improved understanding of sleep alterations may affect clinical management and anticipatory guidance at discharge from the neonatal units.

SCORING METHODS

Depending on the drug exposure experienced by each infant, the time frame for withdrawal can vary. Most experts agree that monitoring for at least 72 to 120 hours after birth is sufficient to recognize the symptoms of withdrawal, although with long-acting opioids in particular, such as methadone, the withdrawal period can be longer.[7]

Several scoring tools are available for measuring signs and symptoms of withdrawal and to determine when to start therapy, based primarily on observations from opioid withdrawal.[44] The most commonly used scale in the United States is the modified Finnegan Neonatal Abstinence Scoring system (**Fig. 1**).[7,45] This comprehensive tool is completed every 4 to 6 hours with items covering central nervous system, autonomic, vasomotor, and gastrointestinal signs and symptoms. In a study of normal newborns, the average Finnegan score at days 1 to 3 of life was 2, but variation occurred up to a 95th percentile of 7, therefore scores of 8 or higher were considered pathologic.[46] This knowledge that all newborns display some level of Finnegan scoring immediately after birth in comparison with 5 to 6 weeks of life is important when caring for infants with prolonged hospitalizations.[46] A typical protocol is to reevaluate an infant scoring more than 8 within 1 hour, with initiation of medication if the score is consistently high. Other scoring tools are also available, including the Lipsitz Neonatal Drug-Withdrawal Scoring System, the Ostrea tool, the Neonatal Withdrawal Inventory, and the Neonatal Narcotic Withdrawal Index.[6]

NAME:_____   MR#:_____

Nursing Instructions
1. If infant scores >8, rescore in one hour
2. Notify physician if two scores, 1 hour apart, >8
3. Give medication as prescribed by physician every 3-4 hours. Do not exceed 4 hours in dosing.

Initiation of morphine sulfate therapy:

CATEGORIES	SCORE	Morphine= Morphine Sulfate oral solution
0	0-8	0 0.4 mg/ml
I	9-12	0 .04 mg
II	13-16	0.08 mg
III	17-20	0.12 mg
IV	21-24	0.16 mg
V	>=25	0.20 mg

SIGNS AND SYMPTOMS	SCORE	Date /time	Date /time	Date /time	Date /time	Date /time	Date /time	Date /time	Date /time	Date /time	Date /time	Date /time	Date /time
Excessive Cry	2 - 3												
Sleeps < 1 hour after feeding	3												
Sleeps < 2 hours after feeding	2												
Sleeps < 3 hours after feeding	1												
Hyperactive Moro Reflex	1												
Markedly Hyperactive Moro Reflex	2												
Mild Tremors: Disturbed	1												
Moderate-Severe Tremors: Disturbed	2												
Mild Tremors: Undisturbed	1												
Moderate-Severe Tremors: Undisturbed	2												
Increased Muscle Tone	1-2												
Excoriation (specific area)	1 - 2												
Generalized Seizure	8												
Fever > 37.2 C	1												
Frequent Yawning	1												
Sweating	1												
Nasal Stuffiness	1												
Sneezing	1												
Tachypnea (Respiratory Rate> 60/min)	2												
Poor Feeding	2												
Vomiting	2												
Loose Stools	2												
Failure to Thrive (weight gain ≥ 10% below birth weight)	2												
Excessive Irritability	1 - 3												
TOTAL SCORE / CATEGORY													
INITIALS													

Fig. 1. Modified Finnegan scoring system. (*From* Jansson LM, Velez M, Harrow C. The opioid exposed newborn: assessment and pharmacologic management. J Opioid Manag 2009;5:47–55. *Adapted from* Finnegan L, Connaughton J, Kron R, et al. Neonatal abstinence syndrome: Assessment and management. Addict Dis 1975;2:141–58.)

There are no studies comparing the efficacy or future impact of evaluation and pharmacologic treatment based on the use of each of the scoring methods.[44] There are also no studies comparing outcomes with initiation of therapy at different scoring thresholds. It is important for each institution to establish a standardized system for routine monitoring, scoring, and initiation of therapy that fits the needs of their individual patient population. The subjective nature of the evaluation of some of the signs and symptoms of withdrawal can lead to poor reliability, especially when the examiners are not frequently involved in the care of infants with withdrawal symptoms.

PHARMACOLOGIC TREATMENT

The primary goals of treatment during neonatal withdrawal are to alleviate short-term symptomatology to allow healthy feeding, growth, and maternal bonding. There are severe potential consequences of not initiating treatment, including seizures, severe weight loss, failure to thrive, and possibly death, but ultimately withdrawal is thought to be a self-limited process.[10] At present there are no studies delineating the long-term benefits of treatment. There is also significant heterogeneity in treatment patterns in the United States and internationally, and a need for further research to delineate optimal pharmacologic treatment of neonatal withdrawal.[29] When initiating any opioid therapy, it is important to monitor for oversedation in the infant by careful nursing observation, including monitoring for apnea, and assessment of respiratory rate and oxygen saturation.[47]

Opioid monotherapy is currently the most common pharmacologic treatment for neonatal opioid withdrawal.[6,44] A 2010 Cochrane review found that opioid therapy was superior to supportive care in respect of time to regain birth weight, but resulted in prolonged stay in hospital.[48] This review also found that opioids significantly reduced treatment failure in comparison with diazepam but not in comparison with phenobarbital. In addition, there were insufficient data to recommend treatment with any one opioid over another.[48] A confounding factor in many of these studies was polysubstance abuse, resulting in a post hoc analysis hypothesis by the Cochrane group that infants exposed primarily to opioids may fare better with opioid-only treatment. Despite the cited methodological flaws with many of the studies used for this Cochrane article, opioids are recommended as the first-line therapy in this review as well as by most professional organizations.[7,48]

Historically, NAS was treated with tincture of opium combined with alcohol, or paregoric, a combination of multiple ingredients, several of which are now known to be toxic to infants.[6] Opioids used currently include formulations of morphine, methadone, and, most recently, buprenorphine.[29] Morphine preparations currently in use are short-acting ethanol-free preparations administered every 3 to 4 hours based on their short half-life, although the pharmacokinetics of oral morphine in newborns is unknown and there can be significant interpatient variability.[29] There is currently no evidence or agreement on the optimal oral morphine regimen, or a safe maximum daily dose, although published studies report an average of 0.06 to 0.24 mg/kg/d.[29] The protocol used in the MOTHER trial was not weight based, and instead escalates the dose based on the Finnegan score. The authors have successfully adapted this protocol for use in infants at the University of New Mexico (**Box 3**). Each institution should aim to create or adopt a standardized protocol until more information becomes available.

Methadone's longer half-life presents benefits and challenges when used for neonatal opioid withdrawal. Longer intervals between doses may facilitate outpatient therapy; however, this is accompanied by a longer duration of therapy when used for buprenorphine-exposed neonates,[17] and newborn pharmacokinetics are largely unexplored.[29] According to a 2006 survey, only about 20% of NICUs in the United States were using methadone.[5] There is only one study comparing morphine with methadone for in utero methadone or heroin exposure, with no significant difference in length of stay in hospital.[49] Further studies are needed to determine ideal treatment populations, regimens, and comparisons with other opioid therapies. A sample treatment protocol for methadone therapy in neonatal withdrawal is presented in **Box 4**.

As a novel therapy for neonatal opioid withdrawal, buprenorphine has only limited data. Two recent studies at the same institution have shown that buprenorphine is a safe alternative for treatment of neonatal opioid withdrawal, and resulted in a shorter length of stay when compared with morphine. However, more infants required adjunctive therapy with phenobarbital.[50,51] Further studies are needed before buprenorphine can be used for the treatment of neonatal withdrawal outside of a research setting.

In addition to opioid therapy, several other medications are in use as adjunctive therapy, primarily for infants with persistent severe symptoms after monotherapy with an opioid. Some experts also believe that cotherapy combining an opioid with

---

Box 3
University of New Mexico protocol for short-acting morphine for neonatal opioid withdrawal

Dose given every 3–4 h with feeds; do not exceed 4 h between doses of morphine (0.04 mg/0.1 mL)

A. Score Dose for Initiation (based on modified Finnegan score)

   0–8 None

   9–12 0.04 mg/dose

   13–16 0.08 mg/dose

   17–20 0.12 mg/dose

   21–24 0.16 mg/dose

   25 or above 0.20 mg/dose

B. Score Morphine Initiation

   • If neonate scores 9–12, rescore after feeding or within the hour and if rescore is 9–12, start treatment based on highest score. If rescore is 0–8, do not initiate treatment

   • If initial score is 13 or greater, start treatment immediately without reassessment

C. Morphine Maintenance/Escalation

   • Maintain dose if score 0–8

   • Increase dose by 0.02 if score is 9–12 (rescore before dosing)

   • Increase dose by 0.04 if score 13–16

   • Increase score by 0.06 if score 17–20

D. Weaning Instructions

   • Maintain on dose 48 h before starting weaning

   • Wean 0.02 mg morphine every day for a score of 0–8

   • Defer wean for score 9–12

E. Re-escalation

   • If neonate scores 9–12, rescore as described for initiation

   • If second score is 9–12, increase morphine 0.01 mg every 3–4 h

   • If 2 consecutive scores 13–16, increase 0.02 mg every 3–4 h

   • If 2 consecutive scores 17–20, increase 0.04 mg every 3–4 h, etc

Timing of scoring: Hospitalized infants are scored every 3–4 h before feeds. Reassessment occurs immediately after feeds or within 1 hour.

Oxygen saturation and respiratory rate is assessed 30–60 minutes after first 2 doses and after any dose escalation.

Adapted from Jones HE, Kaltenbach K, Heil SH, et al. Neonatal abstinence syndrome after methadone or buprenorphine exposure. N Engl J Med 2010;363:2320–31.

---

phenobarbital as the initial treatment may be beneficial for infants with polysubstance exposure, but there is currently no consensus of evidence to support this.[29] The only trial examining the effects of initial combination therapy with opioids and phenobarbital demonstrated benefits of shorter hospital stay, less severe withdrawal, and less hospital cost.[52] A recent randomized controlled trial using clonidine as adjunctive therapy demonstrated a shorter length of treatment and less opioid requirement for infants cotreated with clonidine.[53] Adverse outcomes were also seen in this study,

---

Box 4
University of New Mexico methadone protocol for neonatal opioid withdrawal syndrome

Step 1: 0.7 mg/kg/24 h divided into 6 doses (every 4 h) is starting dose

Step 2: Decrease dose by half, which is 50% of starting dose every 4 h

Step 3: Same dose, which is 50% of starting dose every 6 h

Step 4: Same dose, which is 50% of starting dose every 8 h

Step 5: Same dose, which is 50% of starting dose every 12 h

Step 6: Decrease dose by half, which is 25% of starting dose every 12 h

Step 7: Same dose, which is 25% of starting dose every 24 h

Use with nurses' expertise when decreasing doses. Decrease doses based on daily assessment of needs. Each baby is different and will score individually.

If scores are >8 three consecutive times or if the mean score of three consecutive scores is >8 or if the scores are >12 two consecutive times, then continuing present dose and interval may be necessary. Observe for 48 h after last dose. If infant has gained weight rapidly, it may be necessary to adjust dose by using current weight as the basis for calculating the current dose while maintaining the current interval.

Any infant with severe NAS in Level 1 newborn nursery requiring escalation of methadone dose to greater than 0.7 mg/kg/24 h or the addition of clonidine as an adjunctive pharmacologic treatment should be transferred to Level 2 nursery for evaluation and monitoring.

---

including greater rebound withdrawal and need for reinitiation of opioid therapy in the clonidine group, as well as possibly unrelated outcomes of myocarditis and sudden infant death syndrome indicating the need for more observation.[53] In addition, a recent prospective study of adjunctive therapy with an opioid plus clonidine versus phenobarbital found a shorter stay in hospital with phenobarbital, but an overall longer treatment time when compared with clonidine.[54] Additional studies are needed to determine the safety and efficacy of using phenobarbital or clonidine in conjunction with an opioid to decrease withdrawal severity.[55,56] A 2010 Cochrane review of studies on adjunctive therapies concluded that opioid monotherapy remains superior for the treatment of neonatal opioid withdrawal.[56]

NONPHARMACOLOGIC TREATMENT

Box 5 summarizes several aspects of nonpharmacologic therapy that are beneficial for NOWS and should be initiated in any infant at risk.[44] Because infants experiencing withdrawal are hyperarousable and have altered sleep/wake states, ensuring a dark, quiet environment with low stimuli is essential in determining the true need for medications and avoidance of false elevation of scoring. Swaddling, skin-to-skin, pacifiers, and "cluster care" to minimize stimulation are also common practices thought to be beneficial.[57,58]

Several studies have explored complementary and alternative medicine techniques for neonatal withdrawal. Massage therapy and physical therapy can be used to treat hypertonicity and overstimulation.[58] Music therapy has been shown to calm infants and regulate sleep patterns, and lavender aromatherapy and exposure to the mother's scent have been shown to reduce stress and decrease cortisol levels in infants.[58,59] Acupuncture is commonly used for adult detoxification, and the use of acupuncture or acupressure in neonates offers another potential alternative treatment for neonatal withdrawal.[60]

| Box 5 |
| Nonpharmacologic interventions |

Hyperarousability

  Cluster care

  Dark, quiet environment

  Swaddling

  Skin-to-skin

  Music therapy

  Aromatherapy

Hypertonicity

  Physical therapy

  Massage

Mother-Infant Bonding

  Breastfeeding support

  Rooming-in where possible

  Family education

  Maternal opioid maintenance programs

The initial appropriate hospital setting for newborns can vary between institutions and by clinical severity.[47] Possible options for infants at risk for opioid withdrawal include the NICU, an intermediate-care Level 2 nursery, a Level 1 nursery apart from the mother, or rooming-in of baby with the mother in a regular postpartum unit. The practice of rooming-in has been shown in recent studies of neonatal withdrawal to decrease NICU admission, need for treatment, and length of stay, and to increase the likelihood of discharge in the mother's custody.[61,62] Fostering the mother-infant dyad early in the neonatal period through examinations in the mother's room, and teaching mothers to respond to infant behavior, can improve nurturing behaviors crucial to infant development.[63] At the University of New Mexico, infants are routinely admitted to dyad care on the Mother-Baby unit; however, infants requiring escalation of the methadone dosing beyond the initial 0.7 mg/kg/24 hours, the addition of clonidine as adjunctive therapy, or gavage feedings to maintain adequate intake are transferred to the Level 2 nursery or NICU.

The role of breastfeeding in the management of neonatal opioid withdrawal has been the focus of several recent studies. As rooming-in helps support breastfeeding, it can be difficult to elucidate which practice is responsible for the improved outcomes. Buprenorphine and methadone enter breast milk in small amounts, and are considered to be safe regardless of the maternal dose of opioid replacement therapy.[57,64] As buprenorphine is not well absorbed orally, infant exposure through breast milk may be limited to absorption from the oral mucosa. Several studies have demonstrated significant benefits of breastfeeding in neonatal withdrawal, including less requirement for pharmacologic treatment, shorter duration of treatment, and shorter hospital stays, regardless of type of drug exposure or gestational age.[13,22,26,65,66] Most professional organizations including the American College of Obstetricians and Gynecologists,[67] the American Academy of Pediatrics,[68] and the Academy of Breastfeeding Medicine[69] now endorse breastfeeding in neonatal withdrawal if women have been stable on opioid replacement therapy before delivery and there are no other contraindications such as active substance abuse, hepatitis C with nipple trauma, or HIV. It is important to counsel women in the prenatal period and to encourage breastfeeding where appropriate, as many women will encounter guilt regarding their history of substance abuse and may be discouraged by outside parties who are not aware of the benefits of breastfeeding for neonatal withdrawal. In a study in Maine of 85 mother-baby pairs in a long-term buprenorphine program, 76% of women chose to breastfeed, and 66% of these women continued up to 6 to 8 weeks after birth.[65] In addition, breastfed infants had lower peak Finnegan scores and less requirement for pharmacologic therapy than bottle-fed infants in the same group.[65] In a large study in Boston of 276 mother-baby pairs on methadone or buprenorphine, only 24% of eligible mothers attempted breastfeeding at the hospital, and 60% of these women stopped within 1 week.[70] It is therefore important for providers to understand the eligibility and benefits of breastfeeding for neonatal opioid withdrawal, and support mothers who do not have contraindications throughout the initial hospital postpartum period and beyond.

DEVELOPMENTAL AND FAMILY OUTCOMES

There is limited information about the long-term effects of maternal opioid exposure and neonatal opioid withdrawal or treatment on infant development. Confounding factors include exposure to multiple substances, coexisting psychiatric and medical problems in mothers, and the ongoing socioeconomic sequelae of drug abuse. Opioid exposure may alter the development of synaptic connections and lead to problems with maturation of signaling circuitry.[71] Prenatal opioid exposure may also cause neurochemical and neurobehavioral adaptation in the fetal brain to achieve neurotransmitter signaling homeostasis, and result in interruption of normal brain function with long-term deficits.[71] Efforts to regulate in the μ-opioid receptor systems, the serotonin system, and the dopamine system become evident after delivery with loss of exogenous opioid. Withdrawal symptoms represent the earliest abnormalities in the infant responding to an environment without exogenous opioids until replacement treatment begins if needed. The combined effects of reregulation after birth or treatment with morphine or methadone may contribute to further developmental concerns. Recent studies comparing well-matched controls with methadone-exposed infants have shown subtle differences in neurocognitive functioning and motor development early in infancy that persist at several months of life.[13,72]

Efforts to characterize effects of prenatal drug exposure on specific brain regions have focused on imaging methods such as volumetric magnetic resonance imaging (MRI), functional MRI and magnetic resonance spectroscopy (MRS), and diffusion tensor imaging (DTI), which provide information about functional, metabolic, and region-specific variations in the brain, respectively. Using these methods, infants with prenatal cocaine and methamphetamine exposure had reduced brain volume in the dopamine neurotransmitter-rich putamen and subcortical areas, suggesting diffuse and long-lasting alterations in the brain.[73] However, functional MRI and MRS studies found possible compensatory processes from injuries caused by prenatal exposure, raising the possibility of developmental and neuroplastic brain recovery.[73] These MRI findings suggest a need for future research examining brain regions that may lead to improved knowledge regarding developmental outcomes for infants with prenatal opioid exposure.

Studies attempting long-term developmental follow-up present multiple challenges, and investigators agree that postnatal environmental factors have a primary impact on early childhood outcomes. However, recent meta-analyses of long-term developmental outcomes came to the clear conclusion that when opioid-exposed infants were compared with opioid-free controls, there was consistent evidence of neurodevelopmental impairment, regardless of the age at testing or the tool used to assess these infants.[74] In an Australian cohort study, opioid-exposed infants had significantly lower scores with all assessment tools used, except for the psychomotor development index of the Bayley Scales of Infant Development. The differences appeared significant for cognitive function at the 18-month assessment persisting to the 3-year assessment measured with the Stanford Binet Intelligence Scale and the Reynell language scales.[74] Social maturity was also significantly lower for opioid-exposed children than for control children at 3 years.[74]

In the context of findings suggesting short-term and long-term challenges to normal infant and early childhood development, it is clear that treatment of mothers in a structured program for opioid dependence is beneficial to the newborn, in comparison with no therapy.[29] Infant outcomes after prenatal opioid exposure may be improved by modifying the biopsychosocial conditions of their parents starting in the newborn period. This process can begin as described herein, with rooming-in and breastfeeding support in units designed to treat neonatal opioid withdrawal where parents may receive professional support in providing the daily health and nurturing activities needed by the infants. Unfortunately, after hospital discharge very little comprehensive long-term medical and mental health care is commonly provided to families for the complicated health issues associated with opioid abuse and neonatal development after opioid withdrawal.

Women with substance-abuse disorders commonly have coexisting mental health disorders, which may worsen in the postpartum period because of an altered hormonal milieu and sleep patterns. This situation may also be exacerbated when their newborns require inpatient care for neonatal withdrawal. Many of the women with dual diagnoses have difficulties with the structure and routines of the inpatient wards, and find themselves in conflict with the professional staff over behaviors such as taking a cigarette break or returning to the unit after leaving the hospital for the drug treatment center to access daily methadone. Experienced hospital staff should meet with the parent and develop a supportive plan for the time the mother can spend on the unit or rooming-in. Long-term prospects for maintaining custody of the child by the mother varies by hospital policies with respect to reporting to the child protection authorities, the clinical decision making around obtaining urine or other body substance drug screens, the availability of drug screens, and medical and forensic interpretation of the results.

AREAS FOR IMPROVEMENT

While there continue to be gaps in scientific knowledge, there are also many gaps in systems and biopsychosocial knowledge of neonatal withdrawal. Only about half of NICUs in the United States have a written protocol for the diagnosis and management of NAS.[5] Nurses working in the NICU also report frustration and burnout from caring for infants with withdrawal, and may underestimate the skill and importance of caring for these newborns.[75] Support of families in the hospital environment while their child undergoes treatment for neonatal opioid withdrawal must address a broader set of needs, foremost among which is the ongoing medication-assisted treatment of the mother on methadone or buprenorphine. Lactation support systems are need to improve breastfeeding rates for opiate addicted women who are considered appropriate candidates to initiate breastfeeding. Many parents who have a history of substance-use disorders also confront insecure housing, inadequate access to food, and lack of transportation. The hospital system and its staff need to understand the challenges parents may face in being present at their child's bedside for the amount of time the unit professionals deem important. Greater consideration of the social, historical, and political influences of society on the medical phenomenon of neonatal abstinence will help strengthen research and improve outcomes for mothers and babies.[76]

REFERENCES

1. Patrick SW, Schumacher RE, Benneyworth BD, et al. Neonatal abstinence syndrome and associated health care expenditures. JAMA 2012;301:1934–40.
2. Substance Abuse and Mental Health Services Administration. Results from the 2012 National Survey on Drug Use and Health: Summary of National Findings, NSDUH Series H-46, HHS Publication No. (SMA) 13-4795. Rockville (MD): Substance Abuse and Mental Health Services Administration; 2013.
3. Havens JR, Simmons LA, Shannon LM, et al. Factors associated with substance use during pregnancy: results from a national sample. Drug Alcohol Depend 2009;99:89–95.
4. Hayes MJ, Brown MS. Epidemic of prescription opiate abuse and neonatal abstinence. JAMA 2012;E1–2. http://dx.doi.org/10.1001/jama.2012.4526. Published online.
5. Sarkar S, Donn SM. Management of neonatal abstinence syndrome in neonatal intensive care units: a national survey. J Perinatol 2006;26:15–7.
6. Jansson LM, Velez M, Harrow C. The opioid exposed newborn: assessment and pharmacologic management. J Opioid Manag 2009;5:47–55.
7. Hudak ML, Tan RC, Committee on Drugs, Committee on Fetus and Newborn, American Academy of Pediatrics. Neonatal drug withdrawal. Pediatrics 2012; 129:e540–60.
8. Cotten SW. Drug screening in the neonate. Clin Lab Med 2012;32:449–66.
9. Jansson LM, Velez M. Neonatal abstinence syndrome. Curr Opin Pediatr 2012; 24:252–8.
10. Behnke M, Smith VC, Committee on Substance Abuse, Committee on Fetus and Newborn. Prenatal substance abuse: short- and long-term effects on the exposed fetus. Pediatrics 2012;131:e1009–24.
11. Bauer CR, Shankaran S, Bada HS, et al. The maternal lifestyle study: drug exposure during pregnancy and short-term maternal outcomes. Am J Obstet Gynecol 2002;186:487–95.
12. Ebner N, Rohrmeister K, Winklbaur B, et al. Management of neonatal abstinence syndrome in neonates born to opioid maintained women. Drug Alcohol Depend 2007;87:131–8.
13. Logan BA, Brown MS, Hayes MJ. Neonatal abstinence syndrome: treatment and pediatric outcomes. Clin Obstet Gynaecol 2013;56:186–92.
14. Finnegan LP. Management of pregnant drug-dependent women. Ann N Y Acad Sci 1978;311:135–46.
15. Lejeune C, Simmat-Durand L, Gourarier L, et al. Prospective multicenter observational study of 260 infants born to 259 opiate-dependent mothers on methadone or high-dose buprenorphine substitution. Drug Alcohol Depend 2006;82:250–7.
16. Jones HE, Johnson RE, Jasinski DR, et al. Buprenorphine versus methadone in the treatment of pregnant opioid-dependent patients: effects on the neonatal abstinence syndrome. Drug Alcohol Depend 2005;79:1–10.

17. Jones HE, Kaltenbach K, Heil SH, et al. Neonatal abstinence syndrome after methadone or buprenorphine exposure. N Engl J Med 2010;363:2320–31.
18. Cleary BJ, Donnelly J, Strawbridge J, et al. Methadone dose and neonatal abstinence syndrome—systematic review and meta-analysis. Addiction 2010;105: 2071–84.
19. McCarthy JJ, Leamon MH, Parr MS, et al. High-dose methadone maintenance in pregnancy: maternal and neonatal outcomes. Am J Obstet Gynecol 2005;193: 606–10.
20. Berghella V, Lim PJ, Hill MK, et al. Maternal methadone dose and neonatal withdrawal. Am J Obstet Gynecol 2003;189:312–7.
21. McCarthy JJ, Leamon MH, Stenson G, et al. Outcomes of neonates conceived on methadone maintenance therapy. J Subst Abuse Treat 2008; 35:202–6.
22. Pritham UA, Paul JA, Hayes MJ. Opioid dependency in pregnancy and length of stay for neonatal abstinence syndrome. J Obstet Gynecol Neonatal Nurs 2012; 41:180–90.
23. Lim S, Prasad MR, Samuels P, et al. High-dose methadone in pregnant women and its effect on duration of neonatal abstinence syndrome. Am J Obstet Gynecol 2009;200:70.e1–5.
24. Dryden C, Young D, Hepburn M, et al. Maternal methadone use in pregnancy: factors associated with the development of neonatal abstinence syndrome and implications for healthcare resources. BJOG 2009;116:665–71.
25. Seligman NS, Salva N, Hayes EJ, et al. Predicting length of treatment for neonatal abstinence syndrome in methadone-exposed neonates. Am J Obstet Gynecol 2008;199:396.e1–7.
26. Isemann B, Meinzen-Derr J, Akinbi H. Maternal and neonatal factors impacting response to methadone therapy in infants treated for neonatal abstinence syndrome. J Perinatol 2011;31:25–9.
27. Burns L, Mattick RP, Lim K, et al. Methadone in pregnancy: treatment retention and neonatal outcomes. Addiction 2007;102:264–70.
28. Opioid abuse, dependence, and addiction in pregnancy. Committee Opinion No. 524. American College of Obstetricians and Gynecologists. Obset Gynecol 2012;119:1070–6.
29. Kraft WK, van den Anker JN. Pharmacologic management of the opioid neonatal abstinence syndrome. Pediatr Clin North Am 2012;59:1147–65.
30. Jones HE, Dengler E, Garrison A, et al. Neonatal outcomes and their relationship to maternal buprenorphine dose during pregnancy. Drug Alcohol Depend 2013; 134:414–7.
31. O'Connor AB, O'Brien L, Alto WA. Are there gender related differences in neonatal abstinence syndrome following exposure to buprenorphine during pregnancy? J Perinat Med 2013;41:621–3.
32. Holbrook A, Kaltenbach K. Gender and NAS: does sex matter? Drug Alcohol Depend 2010;112:156–9.
33. Doberczak TM, Kandall SR, Friedmann P. Relationship between maternal methadone dosage, maternal-neonatal methadone levels, and neonatal withdrawal. Obstet Gynecol 1993;81:936–40.
34. Gaalema DE, Heil SH, Badger GJ, et al. Time to initiation of treatment for neonatal abstinence syndrome in neonates exposed in utero to buprenorphine or methadone. Drug Alcohol Depend 2013;113:266–9.
35. Oei J, Lui K. Management of the newborn infant affected by maternal opiates and other drugs of pregnancy. J Pediatr Child Health 2007;43:9–18.

36. Iqbal MM, Sobhan T, Ryals T. Effects of commonly used benzodiazepines on the fetus, the neonate, and the nursing infant. Psychiatr Serv 2002;53: 39–49.

37. Sanz EJ, De-las-Cuevas C, Kiuru A, et al. Selective serotonin reuptake inhibitors in pregnant women and neonatal withdrawal syndrome: a database analysis. Lancet 2005;365:482–7.

38. Moses-Kolko EL, Bogen D, Perel J, et al. Neonatal signs after late in utero exposure to serotonin reuptake inhibitors: literature review and implications for clinical applications. J Am Med Assoc 2005;293:2372–83.

39. Wachman EM, Newby PK, Vreeland J, et al. The relationship between maternal opioid agonists and psychiatric medications on length of hospitalization for neonatal abstinence syndrome. J Addict Med 2011;5:293–9.

40. Choo RE, Huestis MA, Schroeder JR, et al. Neonatal abstinence syndrome in methadone-exposed infants is altered by level of prenatal tobacco exposure. Drug Alcohol Depend 2004;75:253–60.

41. Wachman EM, Hayes MJ, Brown MS, et al. Association of OPRM1 and COMT single-nucleotide polymorphisms with hospital length of stay and treatment of neonatal abstinence syndrome. JAMA 2013;309:1821–7.

42. Spitzmiller RE, Morrison T, White R. Babies with neonatal abstinence syndrome have electrographic seizures and altered sleep on amplitude-integrated EEG. Neonatol Today 2013;8:1–7.

43. O'Brien CM, Jeffery HE. Sleep deprivation, disorganization and fragmentation during opiate withdrawal in newborns. J Paediatr Child Health 2002;38:66–71.

44. Grim K, Harrison TE, Wilder RT. Management of neonatal abstinence syndrome from opioids. Clin Perinatol 2013;40:509–24.

45. Finnegan LP, Connaughton JF Jr, Kron RE, et al. Neonatal abstinence syndromes: assessment and management. Addict Dis 1975;2:141–58.

46. Zimmermann-Baer U, Nötzli U, Rentsch K, et al. Finnegan neonatal abstinence scoring: normal values for first 3 days and weeks 5-6 in non-addicted infants. Addiction 2010;105:524–8.

47. Dow K, Ordean A, Murphy-Oikonen J, et al. Neonatal abstinence syndrome: clinical practice guidelines for Ontario. J Popul Ther Clin Pharmacol 2012;19:e488–506.

48. Osborn DA, Jeffery HE, Cole MJ. Opiate treatment for opiate withdrawal in newborn infants. Cochrane Database Syst Rev 2010;(10):CD002059.

49. Lainwala S, Brown ER, Weinshenk NP, et al. A retrospective study of length of hospital stay in infants treated for neonatal abstinence syndrome with methadone versus oral morphine preparations. Adv Neonatal Care 2005;5: 265–72.

50. Kraft WK, Gibson E, Dysart K, et al. Sublingual buprenorphine for treatment of neonatal abstinence syndrome: a randomized trial. Pediatrics 2008;122:e601–7.

51. Kraft WK, Dysart K, Greenspan JS, et al. Revised dose schema of sublingual buprenorphine in the treatment of neonatal opioid abstinence syndrome. Addiction 2011;106:574–80.

52. Coyle MG, Ferguson A, Lagasse L, et al. Diluted tincture of opium (DTO) and phenobarbital versus DTO alone for neonatal opiate withdrawal in term infants. J Pediatr 2002;140:561–4.

53. Agthe AG, Kim GR, Mathias KB, et al. Clonidine as an adjunct therapy to opioids for neonatal abstinence syndrome: a randomized, controlled trial. Pediatrics 2009;123:e849–56.

54. Surran B, Visintainer P, Chamberlain S, et al. Efficacy of clonidine versus phenobarbital in reducing neonatal morphine sulfate therapy days for neonatal

abstinence syndrome. A prospective randomized clinical trial. J Perinatol 2013; 33(12):954–9.

55. Beaulieu MJ. Oral clonidine in the management of acquired opioid dependency. Neonatal Netw 2013;32:419–24.

56. Osborn DA, Jeffery HE, Cole MJ. Sedatives for opiate withdrawal in newborn infants. Cochrane Database Syst Rev 2010;(10):CD002053.

57. Jansson LM, Choo R, Velez ML, et al. Methadone maintenance and breastfeeding in the neonatal period. Pediatrics 2008;121:106–14.

58. Sublett J. Neonatal abstinence syndrome: therapeutic interventions. MCN Am J Matern Child Nurs 2013;38:102–7.

59. Field T, Field T, Cullen C, et al. Lavender bath oil reduces stress and crying and enhances sleep in very young infants. Early Hum Dev 2008;84:399–401.

60. Raith W, Kutschera J, Muller W, et al. Active ear acupuncture points in neonates with neonatal abstinence syndrome (NAS). Am J Chin Med 2011;39:29–37.

61. Abrahams RR, Kelly SA, Payne S, et al. Rooming-in compared with standard care for newborns of mothers using methadone or heroin. Can Fam Physician 2007;53:1722–30.

62. Abrahams RR, MacKay-Dunn MH, Nevmerjitskaia V, et al. An evaluation of rooming-in among substance-exposed newborns in British Columbia. J Obstet Gynaecol Can 2010;32:866–71.

63. Velez M, Jansson LM. The opioid dependent mother and newborn dyad: non-pharmacological care. J Addict Med 2008;2:113–20.

64. Pritham UA. Breastfeeding promotion for management of neonatal abstinence syndrome. JOGN Nurs 2013;42:517–26.

65. O'Connor AB, Collett A, Alto WA, et al. Breastfeeding rates and the relationship between breastfeeding and neonatal abstinence syndrome in women maintained on buprenorphine during pregnancy. J Midwifery Womens Health 2013;58:383–8.

66. Abdel-Latif ME, Pinner J, Clews S, et al. Effects of breast milk on the severity and outcome of neonatal abstinence syndrome among infants of drug-dependent mothers. Pediatrics 2006;117:1163–9.

67. ACOG Committee on Health Care for Underserved Women, American Society of Addiction Medicine. Opioid abuse, dependence, and addiction in pregnancy. Committee Opinion No. 524. Obstet Gynecol 2012;119:1070–6.

68. Section on Breastfeeding. Policy statement: breastfeeding and the use of human milk. Pediatrics 2012;129:e827–41.

69. Academy of Breastfeeding Medicine Protocol Committee, Jansson LM. ABM clinical protocol #21:Guidelines for breastfeeding and the drug dependent woman. Breastfeed Med 2009;4:225–8.

70. Wachman EM, Byun J, Phillipp BL. Breastfeeding rates among mothers of infants with neonatal abstinence syndrome. Breastfeed Med 2010;5:159–64.

71. Lester BM, Kosofsky B. Effects of drugs of abuse on brain development. Neurobiology of mental illness. 3rd edition. New York: Oxford University Press; 2009.

72. Marcus J, Hans SL, Jeremy RJ. A longitudinal study of offspring born to methadone-maintained women. Effects of multiple risk factors on development at 4, 8, and 12 months. Am J Drug Alcohol Abuse 1984;10:195–207.

73. Derauf C, Kekatpure M, Neyzi N, et al. Neuroimaging of children following prenatal drug exposure. Semin Cell Dev Biol 2009;20:441–54.

74. Hunt RW, Tzioumi D, Collins E, et al. Adverse neurodevelopmental outcome of infants exposed to opiate in utero. Early Hum Dev 2008;84:29–35.

75. Murphy-Oikonen J, Brownlee K, Montelpare W, et al. The experiences of NICU nurses in caring for infants with neonatal abstinence syndrome. Neonatal Netw 2010;29:307–13.
76. Marcellus L. Neonatal abstinence syndrome: reconstructing the evidence. Neonatal Netw 2007;26:33–40.

Index

Note: Page numbers of article titles are in **boldface** type.

Obstet Gynecol Clin N Am 41 (2014) 335–342
http://dx.doi.org/10.1016/S0889-8545(14)00028-X
0889-8545/14/$ – see front matter © 2014 Elsevier Inc. All rights reserved.

obgyn.theclinics.com

Moving?

Make sure your subscription moves with you!

To notify us of your new address, find your **Clinics Account Number** (located on your mailing label above your name), and contact customer service at:

Email: journalscustomerservice-usa@elsevier.com

800-654-2452 (subscribers in the U.S. & Canada)
314-447-8871 (subscribers outside of the U.S. & Canada)

Fax number: 314-447-8029

Elsevier Health Sciences Division
Subscription Customer Service
3251 Riverport Lane
Maryland Heights, MO 63043

*To ensure uninterrupted delivery of your subscription, please notify us at least 4 weeks in advance of move.

Printed and bound by CPI Group (UK) Ltd, Croydon, CR0 4YY

03/10/2024

01040489-0018